# Just Chaaa...

## Breathing, Feeling, and Touching
## Your Way to More Energy

David Kearney, OMD

*This book is dedicated to the memory of my mother for giving me unwavering love and devotion and for showing me the way in life, and to the memory of my father whose early departure set me on a path that spurred my passion for alternative health.*

Published by Chaaa Healing Media

www.PowerHealing.com

ISBN-13: 978-1515079552
ISBN-10: 1515079554

# Table of Contents

*(cont.)*

*(cont.)*

# CHAPTER ONE
## *You Can Do It*

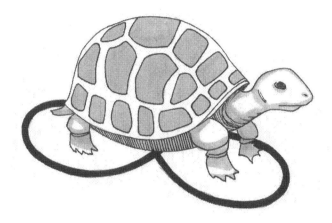

Breath is power! When I refer to the power of breath, I am speaking not only to the power of inhaling and exhaling, but also to the power of the breaths we shape, the songs we sing, the words we speak, and the stories we tell about ourselves and others.

### Breathing Away a Lifelong Stutter

Most people take speaking for granted, but my experiences as a child and adolescent ensured that I do not. I suffered from a chronic stammer so that whenever I was nervous, my words got stuck in my throat and my whole body became tense. The more I tried to speak, the more I locked up. Simple expression was a major embarrassment. In hopes of ridding myself of this affliction, I spent years seeing therapists in Dublin, London, and Sydney.

At the age of twenty and hoping to find relief, I signed up for a course advertised on a poster I saw in the London subway: "How to Win Friends and Influence People," the sign read. It was a Dale Carnegie course in communications and public speaking. I decided to go.

Two hundred or so people wanting to refine their public speaking skills packed the room for the first night, and we were asked to come up the microphone and say our names then spend 20 seconds describing ourselves to the group. This was my worst nightmare, but I was determined to participate and positioned myself so I was among the last to speak.

It was finally my turn to stand in front of hundreds of strangers with only a microphone between me and them. I had rehearsed in my head several times what to say, and the moment of truth had arrived. I stepped up to the microphone, paused for as long as possible, and I then began, but my throat seized shut and allowed only clots and shards of sound to escape. It took me nearly two minutes to get through speaking my name. My plight caught everyone's attention by complete surprise. At long last, the instructor walked up, gently put his hand on my shoulder, and acknowledged me for showing great courage.

The entire class gave me a standing ovation, even though I could not say a word. By the end of the evening, I had been named the most improved speaker and given a Dale Carnegie pen.

I attended eight of the nine course sessions, each time with the same result. I would look around the room, my mind studying the crowd as my body tried to speak. In some strange way, I found it very interesting to observe the audience as they observed me. Some felt embarrassed, some felt compassion. Some other people seemed embarrassed for me while others stifled guffaws or laughed out loud, and others still seemed unsure how to react.

Initially, I was willing to endure almost any amount of embarrassment if it might help me. But when it was time for the final course session, I couldn't bring myself to go anymore. It was too painful. I felt like a freak.

Luckily the zodiac turns and we turn with it and another chance for me to work on my stammer came to me. At the age of 23, an Indian meditation teacher introduced me to a rhythmic breathing technique. After practicing it for only a week, my lifelong stammer disappeared and has not come back. I was astonished that rhythmic breathing could eradicate a problem that traditional therapy had not been able to affect.

Shortly after that, I was invited to join the faculty at the Acupuncture College of Australia, where speaking in front of people would be a daily activity. Because I was so inspired by my new form of breathing and had already made such an improvement in myself, I accepted the position. To my surprise, public speaking—once my greatest fear—became joyous.

I was so impressed by the change in myself that, shortly after I lost my stammer, I became a monk. For five years, I lived a monastic, celibate life, spending many days meditating on my breath. My journey eventually took me to the US where I was invited to lead the Acupuncture department at the California Acupuncture College in Los Angeles. Once again, I was speaking in front of students with not even a hint of a stutter. Some days I taught two three-hour classes, and I still maintained a private practice. Later, I took time off from my academic career and became the private acupuncturist for my guru, Guru Ji, and I traveled extensively, living in ashrams all around the world.

When I ended my devotional service to my guru, I realized that no man is an island and no one has exclusivity on becoming a guru. I returned to the road as an acupuncturist, but this time with some of the most famous rock-n-roll artists of all time. Over the next 15 years I accompanied huge acts on grueling national and international tours. In a short time I went from being unable to speak clearly, to public speaking, to living in meditative ashrams, to attending rock shows almost every night.

Through these experiences, I have come to clearly appreciate the immensely positive impact that conscious rhythmic breathing has on all of us—from rock stars to stutterers to gurus.

It doesn't matter who you are or what issues you might have—everyone can benefit from the breath's life-changing effects. Conscious breathing is a moment-to-moment fusion of nature's medicine, no matter what you desire to heal in yourself.

In order to assimilate the mind-body connection necessary to healing, we must embrace the concept of listening to our bodies rather than always listening to our minds. There is no better way to do that than through conscious breathing.

## Activate Your Healing Powers

When the mind can hear the body without judging it, the mind and body become a team, and that allows us to change the habits that sabotage our well-being. The process begins with listening to your own body. For many people, it is one thing to hear this as an adage, yet quite another to know how much this simple phrase can really mean: *Listen to your body.*

It is easy to hear your body when your temples are throbbing and a headache is pounding against your skull, but it is more difficult when you are facing a general sense of fatigue, the blues, the blahs, or even when you are very angry. It takes practice to begin to listen to your body again, especially when you have been tuning it out for years.

Our ability to listen to our body's intelligence is potent and real, and there is actually nothing obscure or mysterious about it. I have learned this over the course of 35 years of clinical experience and teaching the healing process. I also know that when we ignore our bodies, we shorten our lives. Fortunately, the opposite is also true. If we listen, we can receive specific guidance about what will make each of us live longer and more happily. Just below the surface is a current of health and energy that is ours to harness. The process of tapping into your full energy source is completely possible—it is as simple as breathing.

*"Nature performs the cure, the physician takes the fee."*
– Benjamin Franklin

## The Power of Healing Is Within You

What heals you but you? The healing process that goes to work the instant we get a scrape is carried out by the same body intelligence that causes our hearts to beat and our hair to grow. The natural regenerative systems in the body are making physiological changes every second.

When your body is at its optimum, you do not even have to think about the healing process. On the surface, it appears simple, but even in today's high tech world, the most advanced supercomputers cannot carry out the work that the body engages in on a regular basis.

The healing power within all of us is innate. The body is composed of more than 30 trillion cells. These cells work collectively to make a healthy person, but if those cells become damaged, exhausted, or overworked, the body begins to burn out. The process of reversal is twofold. Initially we must recognize the pattern that has created the imbalance in the first place and then alter it. This might be a pattern of shallow breathing, holding your breath when you're under duress, not eating right, missing meals, or engaging in stressful thinking (i.e., making up stories in our heads after the moment has passed). Or it might be a pattern of feeling underappreciated or unloved, or of refusing to rest even with the knowledge that sleep's restorative powers are paramount to our health.

Every day I give my patients simple and specific healing methods that they can use to maximize their physical and mental well-being. They learn to become aware of their energy-draining habits and to replace them with habits that promote vibrant health. You can do this too!

# The Story of *Chaaa*...

One day I was performing acupuncture on a patient. Once I had inserted all the needles, I told him to just relax. In his English accent, he responded "What do mean, 'just relax'? You bloody well just relax!"

Of course he was joking, but I realized in that moment that telling someone to relax is like telling someone to turn blue. It does not work.

Suddenly, the word "chaaa" appeared to me as an alternative to telling him to relax. "Okay," I then said to him, "just chaaa..."
We both laughed, but it worked, and this new word was born into the English language.

My new submission then, for the Oxford Dictionary, by means of christening the word, is thus:

> **Chaaa** *verb /chah/ 1) The action of releasing body tension through focused breathing and an upright posture without thought interference; 2) (Slang) as in, "Just chill, man!"*

The term has already spread further than its use with my patients. I had been treating a pre-teen patient for a while, and one day his mother came in laughing about an incident that occurred on the road while she was shuttling her son and a group of his friends. The kids had gotten into a debate about something and, as the tension grew, one of my patient's friends called out, "Everybody just chaaa!" At the time, I had already been working on this book and was looking for a unique title for it. Her story gave it to me!

Both of these stories about chaaa involve a lot of laughter, but chaaa is no joke. By practicing it, you will likely spend a lot less time at the doctor's office and will laugh all the way to your body's restorative bank. Not only that, you will earn the best interest rate on your life's energy.

Welcome to chaaa!

*"This is a program about getting things moving."*
– Ringo Starr, from Dr. Kearney's DVD, Power Healing

## Add Chaaa to Your Routine

Committing to a healthy daily routine is essential for living a long life of true abundance. It is the necessary ingredient in maintaining and enjoying your youthful nature.

When you take a little time during the course of your hectic day to rest and rebuild, it is like taking a step backward to go miles forward. This daily approach emphasizes pacing yourself for the long haul. Your routine will incorporate three aspects of chaaa: breath, alignment, and healing touch.

Incorporating chaaa into your life means exercising your awareness. If this is new for you, be patient with yourself. But stay with it, and your new routine will become second nature as you joyously add quality years to your life. As soon as these exercises become new habits, you will begin to experience their benefits.

## How to Use This Book

All of the practices in this book can be used throughout the course of the day. Read them all and find those that resonate with you, and then perform them on a routine basis. Consider them to be as vital as any other regular activity you perform, like brushing your teeth, driving your car, eating food, drinking water, or grocery shopping.

The explanations and theories in this book will help you understand the foundational principles of chaaa, but applying the practices is the real key to unlocking the healing power within you. The practices are simple and your body will quickly adapt to these powerful methods. With practice, they can become new, healthy habits. Give them a try and, after only one month, your life can be forever changed in an amazing way. Your body wants to return to health, to its natural state of chaaa.

# CHAPTER TWO
## *Stress*

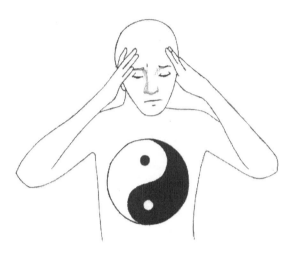

> *"Water is fluid, soft, and yielding. But water will wear away rock,*
> *which is rigid and cannot yield. As a rule, whatever is fluid, soft,*
> *and yielding will overcome whatever is rigid and hard.*
> *This is another paradox: what is soft, is strong."*
>
> – Lao-Tzu (600 B.C.)

Because stress permeates our everyday lives, it's worthwhile to look at it and how it affects our breathing, our posture, and ultimately our health. Let us talk about the Chinese and Western concepts of stress and its treatment.

Yin and yang are the primary energies referred to in Chinese medicine. These words describe everything in nature as binary opposites. Yin is night, and yang is day. Yin is female, and yang is male. Yang represents fire, while yin represents water. Yang is hot; yin is cold. Yang is fast, so, naturally, yin is slow. Yin represents the inside of the body, the organs, and their systems, and yang represents the outside, the musculoskeletal system.

As a living being, you represent the primal spark of yin and yang when the sperm and the ovum, the two fundamental energies of life, come together. The sperm represents yang—the energy that gets us up in the morning and takes us through an active day.

When we are upright, yang energy circulates throughout the muscles, joints, and structure. The heart and the lungs are activated, which engages and directs the circulatory process into the musculoskeletal system. The ovum symbolizes the yin power. We replenish this yin power when we are passive, especially while lying down, meditating, or sleeping. When we are in a yielding state, circulation withdraws from the muscles and is directed toward the organs and inner systems. Good health and long life is a balance between yin and yang.

Today's aggressively competitive society is most definitely dominated by yang. Society has gotten a lot faster and demands exponentially higher expectations. Most people in the Western world now encounter over 100 times more sensory input over the course of 24 hours than those who lived 100 years ago. Chances are, your great-great-grandmother never flew on an airplane, and although she may have traveled by ship, life passed at a slower clip. What has remained the same, however, between you and your great-great-grandmother is physiology. Because our physiology changes much more slowly than the way we live does, as we pick up the pace of our lives, our intense, fiery yang energy can burn out.

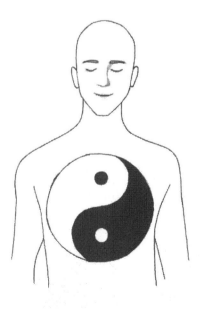

The yin and yang of health is also analogous to the way we use money. Yang is like spending while yin is like saving. Sometimes our energetic generosity or ambition is too large for our pockets, thus inviting debt. In the world of credit cards, we overextend our yang energy. The result is that most of us need to regularly "yin-ify" (i.e., cut down on our use of credit or cut up all of our credit cards and channel money directly back into our bank accounts). When we apply this to our bodies by conserving energy rather than overspending it, we build a greater interest rate on our energy—we not only save it, but we also regenerate our energy. When you can transition from a fast-paced yang lifestyle and slow down into a more restful yin-like state, you can create balance in your life, the perfect complement of yin and yang.

Of course, a certain amount of stress is absolutely necessary in life. This book offers breathing and healing tools that will help you handle the stress effectively instead of being negatively manhandled by it.

## The Yin and Yang of the Nervous System

Think of the autonomic nervous system as Western medicine's version of yin and yang. The autonomic nervous system separates into the parasympathetic and sympathetic nervous systems. The parasympathetic nervous system is yin in this analogy, restful and restorative, while the sympathetic nervous system is yin's active counterpart, yang.

When our brain initiates a fear message, real or imagined, the sympathetic nervous system reacts by releasing stress hormones. The stress reaction supersedes all other systems in the body. Almost immediately there is a reaction: Nerve excitation and stress hormones are released into the blood stream from various sites in the body. Blood flows to the heart and lungs and also to specific muscles. Even our pupils dilate so we can see more. Our sensory systems become very alert.

Here's an example: All of a sudden, on a windy day, the door slams shut and you jump out of your skin. Your primitive reptilian brain comes into play. The sympathetic nervous system regulates stress reactions in your body, akin to the flight, fight, or freeze reaction.

From nature's point of view, we can also see that the sympathetic nervous system hunts for food and the parasympathetic nervous system digests it, supplying the body with energy derived from the hunt.

Figuratively speaking, the parasympathetic nervous system controls the factory of life: immunity, digestion, bone-making, relaxation; in other words, the parasympathetic nervous system— the yin energy—is what makes us feel safe. More than ever, we humans are in a low-grade state of fight or flight, which redirects energy from the internal organs to the guarded muscles. And though our bodies tell us to fight or take off, societal rules dictate that we freeze and tense up these ancient reflexes. As a result, we end up spinning our mental wheels, always ready for something to happen that never does.

This state of being frozen is overwhelmingly prevalent in today's society. I call it "the drop that wears the rock away." Later we will go into these common "freeze states" and how to manage them.

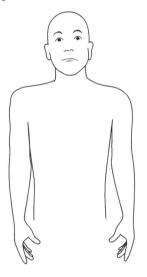

The body is well designed to take short amounts of stress. However, prolonged stress siphons away energy from the parasympathetic nervous system, which is precisely what you need most in order to heal from your stress. In nature, a normal stress cycle runs about 20 minutes in length. From an evolutionary standpoint, that is approximately the amount of time that our bodies need to escape from, and then process, whatever threat exists.

Good health incorporates a healthy balance of sympathetic and parasympathetic nerve response. The value of quickly reverting from sympathetic to parasympathetic nerve functions or from yang to yin is immeasurable. When the danger is over, it is time to breathe easily again, and that is when the body engages the parasympathetic nervous system—yin.

## The Yin and Yang of Active and Passive Breathing

Let's call active breathing "yang breath" and passive breathing "yin breath." Good health is balanced between yin and yang, slow and fast, passive and aggressive, female and male. Today, our fast-paced yang society where everything is "go, go, go!" speeds up your metabolism, heart, and breath, and leads to the premature exhaustion of your overall energy.

Ultimately, too much yang living will burn us out before our time. If we can balance our yang-dominant habits, especially our breathing, with regular and deliberate slow-down time, we will live longer. And let's not forget our friend the turtle, who breathes and moves slowly. There's another parable most everyone is familiar with as well—that of the tortoise and the hare. Remind yourself often who eventually won that race. In the real animal world, faster-breathing animals actually do live shorter lives. Remember that we too are a part of the animal kingdom, designed to breathe slowly, rhythmically, and live long lives, just like the turtle.

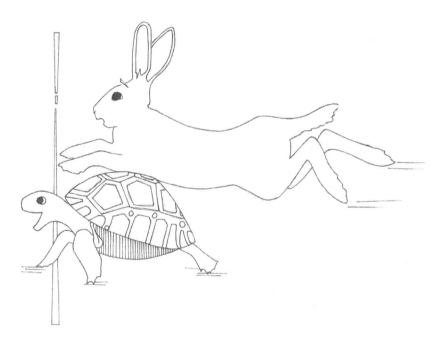

## Modern Day Fight, Flight, or Freeze

Consider our Paleolithic ancestors. When confronted by a saber-toothed cat, the fight-or-flight response kept us alive. Now instead of wild animals, our co-workers and family members are our most common threats. Our bodies respond in a similar fashion, however, acting on that response is no longer acceptable in our society. Take the example of the "mean boss." Your blood is pumping fast, you are nervous and sweaty, but now you have to sit still in a meeting and swallow your fear. Your boss starts yelling at you, and your nervous system is simmering and responds by telling you to fight back or fly away. But since these are no longer socially acceptable options, you smile, hold your breath, and play dead to the great detriment of your health. And the fight-or-flight response now presents us with a different option: freeze.

Ask yourself this question: When was the last time you were attacked by a wild animal or another person or were in some other type of serious danger? In other words, when was the last time you truly needed to either fight for your life or run away to save it? It simply doesn't happen as often as it did for our Paleolithic ancestors.

An overwhelming percentage of our stress is created in our minds as a response to the emotion of fear. Even though a certain amount of fear is normal, beneficial even, we often blow it way out of proportion. We become stuck in our own heads where our fearful thoughts have no escape. The only time we go into our bodies then is when something hurts. Otherwise, there is a disconnection between the mind and body.

Stress is like the constant drip of water that wears away at a rock. The problematic way that modern humans hold onto stress is a constant challenge for the body to cope with.

## The Story of a Frog

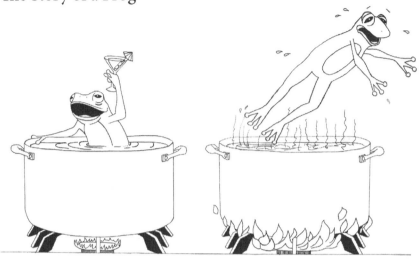

*The simmering water*          *The boiling water*

To see deeper into ourselves, we need only to look into the patterns of nature. For example, when a frog is placed in boiling water, it will quickly jump out. Place this same frog in room temperature water, and the frog will gladly stay in. Yet if you were to slowly increase the temperature, the frog will be unaware of the change, and eventually the boiling water will kill it. This is analogous to the slow, simmering stress that many of us deal with daily, stress that accumulates in both our minds and bodies.

A rock will survive a tidal wave, but it is a steady drop of water that eventually wears through it. Just as a rock survives the tidal wave, we can rely on our strength of character to pull us through periods of personal crises. But it is the chronic stress that sometimes lays dormant in us that will keep us awake at night, that will wear away at us. Ultimately, the drop wears us out. Slow, full body breathing is a way to come out of your head and into your body and reconnect with your whole self.

# Life Is Like a Chick in an Egg

The positive side of our stress comes from the process of freeing ourselves from it, like a chick breaking out of an egg. At first, life is easy; the chick floats around in an ocean of food, absorbing nutrients and essentially eating into a bigger and more developed body. Gradually, it outgrows its shell, so it becomes squished and hungry, and claustrophobia sets in. From this uncomfortable place, the chick begins to struggle. Out of this struggle, the chick develops strong muscles and bones, which allow it to eventually break through its shell and into a whole new world.

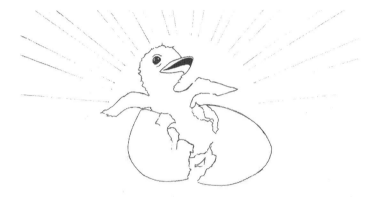

Life's stresses are really just a series of breaking through our shells into the fullness of who we really are. With the right attitude, stress is not only good, it is necessary for healthy growth and survival. It is only when we avoid the stress that is necessary in our lives, thereby creating more of it, that we stay in our shells, forget to breathe, and hold ourselves back. Rather than breaking through the shell into a new beginning, we may try and give in, but when we do that, we tend to invent reasons why life is so difficult.

## *The Two Little Chicks*

Broadly speaking, we can divide people into two categories based on how they deal with stress. I've already mentioned the first of these— this category is full of people who, like the chick described above, grow into bigger bodies and break free. This type of person is not intimidated by life's challenges. Rather than freezing and holding their breath, they breathe through whatever pain comes their way. They are willing to take on the challenge of breaking through their shells. This strengthens them so they can forage for food and function in the world.

The second category is full of those people who struggle. They want to be outside their eggs, but instead of pushing out, they constantly seek external support, hoping someone else will break the egg for them. They rely on alcohol, drugs, or codependent relationships for support, never quite taking full responsibility for their growth. Living this way presents many problems, but a primary one is that if someone breaks the egg prematurely, the chick will die. The chick needs to the feel the hunger and go through the struggle in order to become strong enough to break out from the inside. So there is danger not only in someone else breaking the egg too early but there is also danger in someone else breaking the egg at all. When someone else does that work for us, we do not have the benefit of the growth we were meant to gain from it.

Life and growth are a process of challenges and stresses. Breathing and breaking through progressive shells makes us stronger, allowing for optimal physical and mental growth. It also helps us heal more rapidly when healing is necessary.

## Breathing Is the Way Out

Fortunately, breathing is an incredibly effective adaptive tool that can help you break through any shell. When we slowly, consciously, and rhythmically breathe, we slow down our heart rates, relax our nervous systems, and quickly turn off the fight, flight, or freeze alarm signals; as quickly as it flashes on, the "Fasten Seatbelt" sign blinks off again and choices begin to appear before us. The narrow focus on the problem shifts and our vision expands, allowing us to hold a larger perspective and maintain a calm state during the most stressful of times.

# CHAPTER THREE
## *Healing*

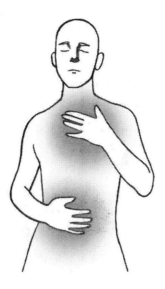

Healing our bodies and healing our minds happens when we connect to our inner selves. Practicing the three steps of healing—optimal breathing, balanced alignment, and healing touch—will help you connect to yourself more deeply. Make them part of your regular routine, and eventually, you will move beyond healing and into a glowing state of health.

## The Three Steps of Healing

### STEP ONE: *Breathing*

Most of us have experienced times when we couldn't breathe. Maybe something got stuck in your throat and blocked your airway, or maybe you were under water and ran out of air. In those situations, your body does everything it can to take a breath. When a person is deprived of air, there is a physical pain in the stomach, and alarms go off all over the body, telling it to breathe. When you can finally take a breath, it is so much better than taking the first bite when you are hungry or taking that first drink when you are thirsty. Those moments when you can't breathe and finally get take a breath make you realize how amazing it is to breathe.

Breathing is your most immediate life energy. It plays a vital role in maintaining good health. Compared to food and water, the other two necessities of life, breathing is much more immediate. It's something we do automatically, and maybe that's why there's very little mainstream information on how to breathe correctly. Whatever the reason, the fact is, in the last 50 years, the public has made major strides in understanding the importance of nutrition. We have also realized the importance of proper hydration. But proper breathing has yet to take its place in the public eye.

When we are born, we do not eat and drink by ourselves—our tiny bodies cannot do it, and we need our parents to feed us. On the other hand, the very first thing our bodies do at birth is fully breathe.

From that day of our first breath, we breathe approximately 23,000 cycles of respiration every single day—that is about 438 cubic square feet of air that passes through us. Within one breath, which takes about five seconds (two seconds in and three seconds out), there are a trillion atoms made up of oxygen, hydrogen, and nitrogen. The oxygen molecule is magnetized to red blood cells and is then carried in the blood through thousands of miles of channels in the body, oxygenating all the trillions of awaiting cells that need that precious air.

### *Observe Your Breath*

Observing your breath throughout the course of the day is the first step to smooth, rhythmic breathing. Most of the breathing methods in this book are exercises that you can perform periodically throughout the day. They facilitate what I call the "constant breath"—that which gets you up in the morning, carries you through breakfast and to your car, pushes you through work, and then takes you back home again. The more you are conscious of the rhythm in each breath, the richer and fuller your life becomes.

There is a subtle but important difference between *experiencing* the feeling of proper breathing and *thinking* about it. The object here is not to think about how your breath feels, but to simply feel it. Through practice, you can learn to allow the experience. This awareness, which I refer to as "being in the body," is important to a successful breathing practice because it facilitates consciously noting the feedback your body gives you. You can start by becoming more aware of what you feel as you breathe—and by allowing any conscious thoughts about it to pass through you.

## EXERCISE: *Observing the Pause*

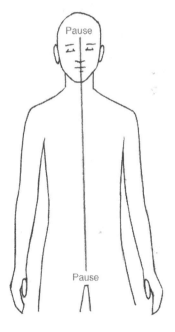

The pause in between breaths is where the yin converges into the yang, and, conversely, where the yang converges into the yin. This pause is a moment of stillness, a neutral point that is neither yin nor yang, neither inhalation nor exhalation. This neutral point is like the calm before the storm. To become even more breath conscious, observe this in-between time. The idea is to feel at both ends of the pause, to notice the difference between the lower pause where the inhalation becomes the exhalation and the upper pause where the exhalation becomes the inhalation.

Begin by breathing normally while lying in a chaaa state. As you focus on your breathing and your body releases tension, focus on the diaphragm muscle spreading beneath your lungs, pulling them downward. At the same time, feel the breath flow down your back, open up your lower back, and then flow into your pelvis and up into your abdomen. Your rib cage and lungs will expand outward.

Follow your inhale all the way to the pause. Observe the pause for a moment—however, avoid forcing the kind of pause that may cause you to hold your breath. Simply be aware that you have drawn in a full inhalation and that your body is full of air and ready to exhale.

As you exhale, your breath moves upward, flowing out through your nose and back into the atmosphere as you arrive at the ascending pause. At that point, you are ready, once again, to receive incoming breath. A normal exhalation is approximately three seconds. A normal inhalation is approximately two seconds. A full, natural exhalation will automatically facilitate a full, natural inhalation. It is a good practice to extend your exhalations. Without forcing or pushing that very last part of your exhale, try to extend it so you can breathe out the lower, heavier waste content of your lungs. Every time we exhale fully, we inhale fully.

The key here is to use the breathing muscles in a relaxed manner so the span of exhalation reaches an extended, natural pause. When your breath is in rhythm, your whole body is physiologically tuned.

### STEP TWO: *Dynamic Alignment*

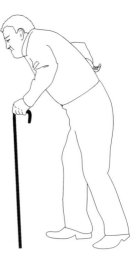

Culturally, we have an image in which the elderly can no longer hold themselves upright without help. Bad posture, however, is one of the main contributors to this traditional symbol of aging. By strengthening our natural powers of alignment, we can keep ourselves from becoming hunched over.

The human eye was designed to look toward the horizon and take in a wide-open space. This design allowed humans to see from afar whether a predator or a meal was present. About 10,000 years ago, humans transitioned from hunters and gatherers to farmers and herders.

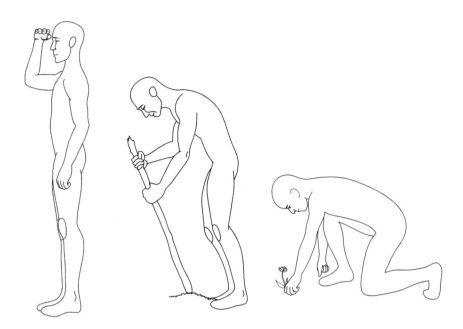

*Humans transitioned from standing upright and looking into the distance
to bending over and looking down at close objects.*

We went from an extended, upright body that looked into the distance,
roaming the plains in search of food, to bending down to see closer
objects in order to dig holes, plant crops, pull weeds, and harvest. We
no longer needed to follow the migrating herds and go
out into the open plains to chase down wild animals. Instead we
became domesticated and started to bend and look down for a living,
which caused our unfortunate change in posture.

Human physical orientation transitioned virtually overnight, if
you look at it from an evolutionary perspective. This change had its
pros and cons—certainly one big pro of evolution has been having
more food and leisure time. We used our free time to build houses,
create new tools and even jewelry. This activity further developed the
dexterity of the thumb and fingers, and this newly found handiwork
led to the sophisticated thumb-and-finger-made world we live in.

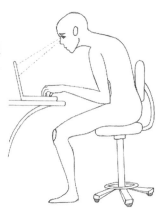

But the major con of the last 10,000 years remains—we modern humans generally bend forward and look down way too much. Other cons include the overuse of poorly crafted chairs and couches. We slouch on the couch and stand and sleep in forward-bending positions, and we sometimes slouch for hours a day working on a computer. Even while walking, many people look down with only occasional glances upward. It took nature millions of years to sculpt a human body designed to extend upward with eyes intended to look outward. And let me remind you that it has only been 10,000 years since humans' physical orientation shifted and we began to bend forward to look down at close objects.

### Bent Forward in Flexion

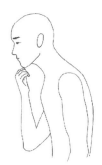

Unless you are lying on your stomach perched up on your elbows with this book in front of you, you are most likely bending forward. Throughout the day, we sit, stand, sleep, and eat in a flexed forward position. When we are concentrating, typically, our heads and shoulders lean forward and our rib cages cave, and that constricts our breathing. In turn, constricting our breath affects our mental states and emotions, not to mention our circulatory and digestive systems. In effect, we are closing in on ourselves, limiting the body's vital functions. To fully inhabit our bodies and cultivate health, we must reverse this tendency toward flexion.

*Head leaning forward concentrating on a thought*

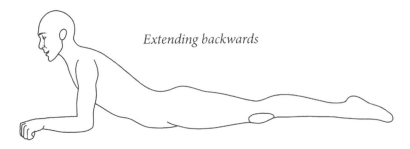

*Extending backwards*

## *Straight Back in Extension*

The opposite and countervailing stretch to flexion is extension, a straighter, even a backward-bending, antidote. Extension creates symmetry within the spinal column as we stretch the frontal muscles of the spine. At the same time, extension loosens the muscles along the back of the spine and helps bring us into a more upright, balanced posture.

By learning to balance properly, modifying your center of gravity, you will redistribute your weight onto your stronger muscles, which helps prevent unnecessary muscle and joint pain. Extension opens up the frontal muscles of the spine because it allows for better circulation, improved organ function, and greater physical comfort and ease. Most importantly, extension lifts the rib cage and opens up the heart— a practice that allows for the fullest and healthiest life experience.

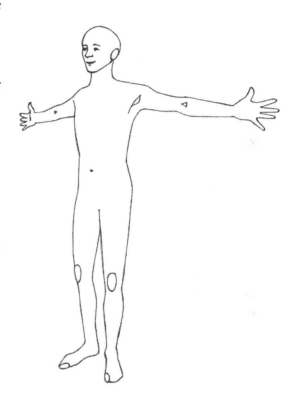

Good posture denotes energetic self-confidence, a physical balance of strength, and an aesthetic sense of grace that others can feel and see. The physical balance principles in this book will literally carry you through life, helping you grow toward alignment and regeneration. It is good to talk about natural alignment but even better to enact it and grow tall toward the clouds.

## STEP THREE: *Healing Self-Touch*

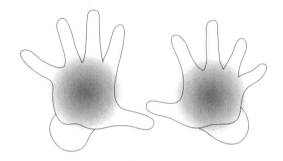

Knowingly or unknowingly, we are all sensualists. In the Western world the subject of self-touch is somewhat taboo because of the sexual implications often associated with it—we have become afraid to touch each other and even ourselves. But touch is not only about sexual stimulation. To be able to heal yourself, you must cross this psychological barrier and be willing to experience a deeper intimacy with yourself through self-touch. You must learn to listen to where your body is asking to be touched and give yourself the healing, loving energy it needs. There is an entire realm of healing that can occur through touch, and you can experience that healing through your hands, your breath, and your intention.

Touch is the ideal medium to transfer energy, and it is the oldest form of communication and healing known to human beings. A gentle touch can single-handedly soothe the nerves, calm emotions, and ease pain. An inherent support mechanism, touch is the body's natural reflex for assisting with an injury, or offering help to a friend in need. Often, people will intuitively press acupuncture points that correlate to their emotional and physical imbalances, such as applying pressure to the forehead to ameliorate depression.

Because the hands can reach any spot on the body's surface, they are perfect tools for releasing blockages and assisting in the process of inner openness.

Accordingly, nature has given special attention to our hands. Enriched with nerves and blood vessels, hands are incredibly sensitive. The hands are powerful receptors that transmit information and energy.

Doctors of Chinese medicine have understood for some 3,000 years that pressing on certain parts of the body relieves pain and treats disease, not only at the site that is being pressed, but in seemingly unrelated areas as well.

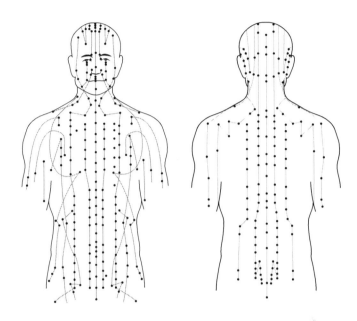

*Some of the many acupuncture points throughout the body.*

How does it work? For centuries doctors have carefully mapped pressure points and the corresponding areas they affect, developing theories about what causes pain and disease and how to treat it.

A central concept involves the flow of chi, or life energy, through the body. Ancient healers of Chinese medicine saw that when they made maps of the body and plotted the location of the points they had pressed to relieve pain, more than 365 principal points appeared to lie along 14 major pathways, or meridians. They theorized that a smooth flow of life energy along those pathways was the key to health and that blockages to that flow caused pain and disease. Touching and breathing into these points directs energy along the meridians.

The newly infused energy can then enter into specific underlying tissues and related organs. Ailing or stagnant organs thus receive the stimulation and support they need to revitalize their functionality.

### Healing Hands

Your healing hands transmit energy, and your underlying circulation gladly receives it. There are many pressure points throughout the body that you can use to get in touch with your own ability to transmit healing energy to yourself. Using these pressure points, you can learn to stimulate circulation in your muscles, joints, and organs with the natural healing power of your hands.

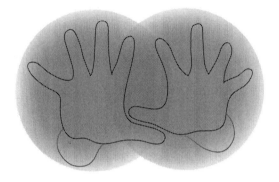

Whether you choose a deeper or a lighter touch, the one thing to remember is that when we touch ourselves, we are touching someone very special indeed. It is the person who has been with you from your first breath, who will stay with you until your last. So when you touch yourself, acknowledge and feel your love for yourself.

By implementing and cultivating the slow breathing, healing touch, and physical alignment practices, you will have them at your disposal for any situation. Developing the habits of slow breathing, maintaining physical balance, and practicing healing touch will radically alter your reactions to your emotional fight, flight, or freeze triggers. These positive habits will significantly de-dramatize the way you experience life's everyday challenges.

## The Reason Turtles Live So Long

There is a Chinese parable that illustrates how the turtle, revered for its lengthy life span, draws its very sustenance from its precious breath. In the tale, a turtle is confined in a cemented underground vault without food and water. Understanding the turtle's secret to longevity, its captors drilled air holes into the cement so that it could breathe. One hundred years later, the vault was re-opened and, to everyone's astonishment, 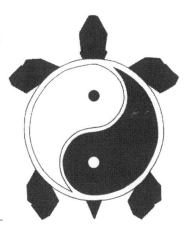 the turtle was very much alive, moving slowly toward the light. Teachers use this tale to explain that breath itself can sustain you. When you recognize its power, you will have the key to eternity.

The importance of breath as a life-giving substance is apparent from the moment of birth. Indeed, it is the most immediate environmental connection we must make in order to survive. When a baby takes that first breath, all of the breathing muscles are fully engaged, and the baby's whole torso expands. Nature makes sure we get it right the first time. Babies are excellent breathers and believe it or not, most adults have forgotten how to breathe like babies. But the good news is that we only need to be reminded.

Breath is also the most direct way to open a connection to your body's natural intelligence. In many cultures, the breath is considered a healing element, even a connection with spirit. Breath is like magic—it feeds, cleanses, and releases energy throughout the body as it circulates. The more we become conscious of our breath, the more we can thoroughly experience life's magic.

### Slow Power

We think we need to be productive, stay active, and get things done. But as we hurry our minds and bodies along, we often just spin our wheels and, in the truest sense, we don't really go anywhere.

Deliberate acts of slowing down during the course of a fast-paced day help set the course for a longer, happier life. We must start by slowing down in the moment and living in the "present tense." It is a matter of bringing yourself into the present, rather than projecting into the future or living in the past. Remember, it is the present moment where everything happens.

There are many ways you can train yourself to slow down and live in the present moment. You might try taking several short breaks to lie down during the day. You might also try simply taking the time to notice what is around you before you jump into a task—you don't have to do anything else but pause, notice what's around you, and breathe.

No matter what activity you're involved in, when you find yourself moving at a rushed pace, deliberately slow down your motion and your breath. This will immediately bring you into the present. The power of now begins with slowing down, and let me remind you again: the race was won by the turtle.

## EXERCISE: *Walking Breath*

> *"You have to stay in shape. My grandmother, she started walking five miles a day when she was 60. She's 97 today and we don't know where the hell she is."*
>
> – Ellen DeGeneres

Walking is how we get around. We walk everywhere—to our cars, our places of work, our bedrooms and meetings. When we are walking in sync with our bodies and in rhythm with our breath, our overall rhythmic balance supports our nervous systems. When we reach our destinations, we are calm, emanating a sense of comfort. Many times, however, we find ourselves running late despite our best intentions. We know we want to replace that rushed internal feeling with a more balanced state, but we are lost in the moment of urgency.

In these cases, I practice the walking breath, and it works for me like a small miracle. Here's how it works: If I am in a hurry and even if I am already late, I deliberately slow my walking way down for about 10 seconds. I feel the rhythm of my slow breath as I move in slow—and I mean turtle-like—motion. As I accelerate back into a regular pace, I notice a change in both my body and my state of mind. A dramatic enhancement can occur within 10 seconds of engaging in this exercise. It is the perfect 10-second step backward that will help you go many miles forward! You can even try it when you're not in a hurry, simply to get your body in tune with a slower rhythm.

## Rest and Be Your Best

Learning how to rest has immeasurable healing advantages. When we rest throughout the day—and that means lying down comfortably, focusing on the breath, and allowing physical and mental tensions to dissolve—our bodies switch from active to passive, and crucial restoration takes place. By stepping away from an external focus and going internal, even briefly, we can reengage with renewed vigor and a sense of inner peace.

You might ask yourself, "If I rest too much, won't it interfere with my sleep?" On the contrary; rest is a stepping stone into sleep. If we do not hone our ability to rest, we do not sleep nearly as well, compromising our vital restorative cycle. Increase your daily rest periods, and your immune, hormonal, and neurological functions will be markedly enhanced.

You also may be thinking, "I can't rest. I have to produce." What you are really saying is that you cannot turn your mind off. The truth is that sleep alone is not enough. And the deeper truth is that we often do not achieve real sleep. We have not retrained our bodies to rest properly. Out of a 24-hour cycle, we are awake, upright, and physically and mentally on the go for 16 hours, allotting only eight of the 24 hours for sleep. Now why not, out of those 16 hectic hours, put aside five to 10 minutes every three hours for rest and focused breathing? This may sound impossible, but don't fret. Fifteen to 30 minutes isn't that much time out of your day, and you will be amazed at the clarity of mind and increased productivity you will experience. It is that one step backward that propels us many miles forward. If you want more out of your daily life, try adding breaks for rest with focused breath to your regimen for just 30 days. Feel free to email me with the results.

### The Power of Slow, Passive, Restful Breathing

My former professor and mentor, Dr. Van Buren, called the
state of slow, passive, restful breathing, "the neutral zone," where we
are neither asleep nor awake, in neutral balance between yin and
yang. This state can be even more beneficial than sleep for health
regeneration—but how can this be so? Because the body is neither
asleep nor awake in this deep, restful, neutral zone, it directs essential
energy to whatever it needs at that particular time. When we access
the deep, restful, neutral state, the body's intelligence automatically
finds its optimal state of being. In this state, an amazing thing happens:
The body produces exactly what we need for a healthier body and
mind. When you access this state, you bring bliss into your life as
well as more energy and better health.

### Resting Before Sleeping

Being aware of your breath not only turns your mind way down, it
facilitates the rest process, which assures a deeper sleep and a more
restful night. In his 2010 book, *The Power of Rest: Why Sleep Alone
Is Not Enough*, Dr. Matthew Edlund cites a handful of studies that
conclude that the general population is sleep deprived. It is a well-
known medical recommendation that we should be receiving eight
hours of restful sleep a night, however most people get far less.
Dr. Edlund also states that, in order to sleep well, you need to
know how to rest.

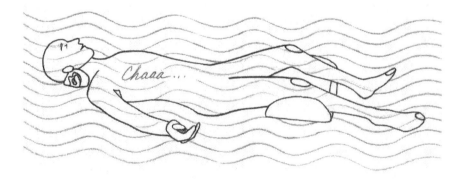

## EXERCISE: *Still Breath Time*

Although all of the breathing practices in this book can be applied at any time or position—standing, sitting, or even running—I have found that lying down and letting the body rest is most fruitful. Restful stillness is conducive to rhythmic breathing. When we are off our feet, our bodies are not using the same energy as when we are upright. When we lie down and mentally and physically let go, the energy is redirected from the external muscles to the internal organs and to their systems (i.e., the immune, digestive, and nervous systems).

To practice still breath time, lie still in a comfortable state with your eyes closed. Consciously release your body tensions and let go. Here again, the trick is to feel it rather than think about it. Feeling your breath is like tasting a drink rather than thinking about tasting it. The message throughout this book is to *feel* rather than *think*.

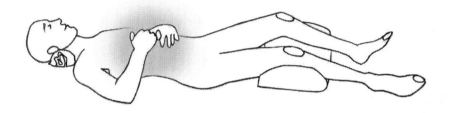

Next, you'll introduce the energy within the still breath. Focus on your normal breath and follow it as it goes in and out. If it is rapid when you begin, just continue to breathe until it returns to a regular pace. This is an easy breath. There is no need to grab or force large doses of oxygen into your lungs. Just chaaa and breathe. Your body will do it for you. It helps to feel or visualize smoothness within your breath and all your breathing muscles.

After a few minutes of this soothing, conscious breathing, you will become aware of the energy within your breath, like a tide going in and out. (This energy is what the Chinese call "essential chi."

Other cultures call it "prana" or "life force.") It is from this energy that you will begin to surf through your body in the waves of breath that will free up areas of obstruction. As you maintain awareness of your chi, your breath will slowly become very still. It will almost seem as if you are barely breathing at all—this is when your body will completely chaaa. You will feel a sense of *being breathed*, as if a soft breeze is blowing through you.

As you consciously breathe in an unforced, smooth breath, the atmosphere fills your entire body. A space opens as you let go, and everything slows down. Your breath is soft and your pulse is smooth. As you drift into stillness, your body becomes weightless. It may seem as if you are not breathing. From this neutral energetic space, we experience a deep letting go and a profound insight into a deeper life source. When we have arrived at that state of deep subliminal rest, our energy is freed to create an overall body/mind balance. We are all designed to access this space on a regular basis. It is amazing how the body and energy systems adapt with the practice of being still and going blissfully into the deeper self.

You may ask yourself if it is really possible for you to reach such a state inside yourself. The answer is absolutely yes—we are all capable of accessing a deep state of inner awareness.

When you have reached this level, you are in the neutral or optimal zone, where actual healing is initiated. It is the optimum balance between yin and yang. This zone is where oxygen and carbon dioxide find a healthy balance and where muscle tension and physical stresses are released. Do not be surprised if, after some practice, you begin to feel a sense of euphoria. This is your body's intelligence thanking you for the energetic nourishment.

## *Energy Tremors*

When the body is in a state of subliminal rest (or deep chaaa), the body often releases energy waves. I think of them as internal earthquakes that send subtle vibrations to create an involuntary rumble or tremor. Tremors occur on a more micro level and are a passive form of releasing energy internally, shaking off or flushing out energetic stagnation. Sometimes, while holding on to physical tension, the body will spontaneously shake, releasing its physical fixations and holding patterns. These energy tremors are part of your body's natural design to move that internal energy flow, bringing with it healing and a wonderful sense of being open from the inside.

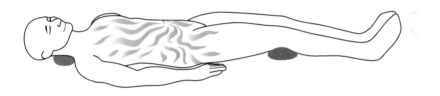

In order to maintain optimum health in this hectic, yang-oriented society of ours, I strongly suggest creating time in your day to yin-ify. Think of it as taking a time *in* instead of a time *out*. Earlier, I referred to this as taking a step backward to go miles forward. For even five minutes—or for an hour a day if you have it—find a way to lie down and slow your breathing. This will allow your body and mind to enter that yin state of subliminal rest and healing. When we retreat internally, we form a balance between yin and yang. The yin state provides the perfect complement to our otherwise yang-dominant mental and physical habits of living in the modern world. It is just another way that the body accesses its healing self. We can condition our bodies to rest even when the going gets hectic. When we rest throughout the course of the day, we naturally yin-ify. We become water instead of that fiery yang tendency that causes our nervous systems to burn out.

## Pulling the Wool over Your Eyes

During a visit to Australia, my brother Bryan took my family to a sheep farm about 50 miles west of Sydney. It was midmorning when we watched an Australian sheep dog guide the sheep to both the right and left, all on a single whistle tone. Later, in his Aussie accent, the farmer told us, "I'm going to show you what it means 'to pull the wool over 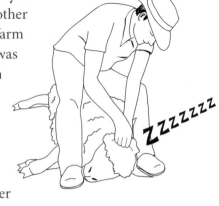 one's eyes.'" With that, he took a piece of wool, placed it over the lamb's eyes, and the lamb fell asleep immediately.

When the farmer removed the wool, the lamb woke up. This was repeated several times, and each time it produced the same result. The saying suddenly became very clear. When we cover our eyes during the day, it may not put us to sleep, but it does put us at ease.

I have flown to Australia to visit family consistently for the past 35 years. After witnessing the sheep relax into sleep, I tried it and found that when I covered my head and closed my eyes, remaining in darkness for as long as possible, I entered a deep state of chaaa.

I tried the technique on the plane to help with jet lag. My normal disorientation caused by jet lag seemed significantly reduced. Try it. The next time you are on a long flight, instead of looking into a laptop or staring at another screen, think about the effect flying is having on your body. You are six miles high, going about 600 miles an hour in an airtight metal container zooming through space. By placing something over your eyes, your body can more easily acclimate.

Even closing your eyes throughout the day is helpful. Coupled with chaaa and focused breath, these methods will minimize the ill effects of everyday life. If you can, cover your eyes and head as well. While covering your head in a public place is not always socially acceptable, society might be mellower if it were.

## EXERCISE: *Cupping Your Hands Over Your Eyes*

Cupping the face has a calming effect on the
nervous system. Rub your hands together briskly
for several seconds to generate some heat. Gently
cup your face and, as you breathe in, visualize the
air flowing into your hands. Exhale, breathing out
through your hands and into your head. Gently
massage your face with the warmth of your hands.
Remember our friend the little lamb who fell fast
asleep when the wool was pulled over his eyes.

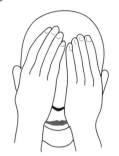

## EXERCISE: *Listening to the Sound of Life*

Begin this exercise by breathing normally while lying in a chaaa
state. When you are prone, your body is not using its energy to stay
upright. When you lie down, you channel that energy to your
internal organs instead.

Placing both hands over your ears, close your eyes and become
aware of the sound of your heartbeat. Listen to the blood flow beneath
your ears as you tune in to your internal soundscape as it creates a
wave-like sound. Breathe deeply into your body. Remain aware of the
sound of both your blood
and breath as you direct your
exhale through your head to
your third eye. Even though
your eyes are closed, there
is an internal light show of
colors and the soundtrack of
your life force dancing with
energy. Most people find this
practice very effective in tuning out the sounds of the outside world
and tuning in to the soundtrack of their own life flow.

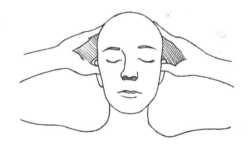

One great way to practice is on your own bed, either before rising
or before sleeping. You can also take a time in during the day on the
couch, floor, or bed. Give yourself about five to 10 minutes and observe
and feel the air flow into your body, then naturally feel it flow back out.

Listen to your breath. Initially, you may experience your "mental mind" butting in and criticizing you. As soon as you recognize this mind involvement, bring your awareness back to the flow of your breath. You are taking time in to listen to the physical sound of your breathing rather than your usual mental chatter. It is like tuning in to a radio station featuring your own natural ocean waves.

As you focus on your breathing and your body lets go in this exercise, pay attention to how your heart rate slows down and your breathing diminishes. Depending on how deep you go, your breath may seem like it has faded into nothingness. In this state, the entire body finds a healthier balance, higher energy, and a deeper state of release. The pH, nervous, hormonal, and immune systems gravitate to an optimal homeostatic balance.

CHAPTER FOUR

# *Breath*

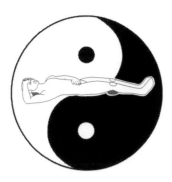

When we encounter problems in our daily lives and seek the advice of friends, we are often told, "Think about it. The answer will come to you." But this keeps your mind locked inside your head. What we really need to hear is this: "Breathe into it."

When we focus our minds on our breathing, we occupy our minds with our life essence. This frees us from those incessant thoughts that spin our wheels and demand attention. As we go about the business of daily life, focused breathing encourages us to "be in it, but not of it." This creates the perfect balance of yin and yang and the ideal remedy to calm a stressed or restless mind.

*"The devil makes work for idle minds."* – Irish proverb

## The Genie in the Bottle

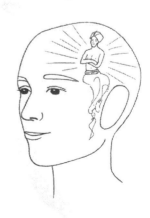

Our minds are like genies in bottles. Around puberty, the genie gets out and we begin to behave like eternally rambunctious teenagers. The genie tells us that it will create anything we desire but adds the caveat, "On one condition—you must always keep me busy." And we say, "Of course!

And now Genie, I want this…" And the genie creates. Sometime later the genie manifests itself again, making something else for us—and the process repeats over and over again. The genie continually comes back and says, "Put me to work. I need to be busy." It will appear while we are asleep, waking us to say, "Give me something to do." The genie becomes angrier with us as we try to take breaks, despite the fact that we spend most of our time trying to keep it busy and happy.

So how do we deal with an angry genie? We tell it to go climb the nearest, tallest tree, and when it gets to the top, to climb down— and when it gets to the bottom, to climb back up. We want the genie to continually go up and down the tree until we need it again.

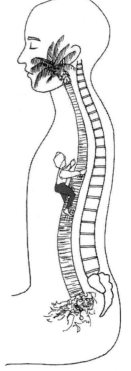

The tree is the breath of life. Just like the genie climbing up and down the tree, when our focus rides the breath in and out, our genie becomes calm and our bodies chaaa.

Conscious breathing is a personal choice. We can choose not to be under the whimsical demands of a restless genie. By simply saying to it, "Hey Genie, take a breath." The busy genie inside you may resist this at first, but by consciously riding the breath in and out, the genie is liberated. A slow, focused, conscious breath frees up the body and mind connection. This brings with it a more total sense of self, clearing the mind's way for a wider mental and emotional perspective.

In over three decades of treating patients, I have found no lines of demarcation separating the mind from the body, nor the body from the mind. So when the mind is locked upstairs in the head, it will eventually become restless. The mind needs to be released into its entire body. Conscious breathing is the very best thing for your genie to do.

## Everyday Breath Riding

To most readily apply the concept of being in the moment, simply focus
on each breath as it passes in and out. It is not possible to entertain
other thoughts simultaneously, while focusing on breathing. Given
that, focused breathing brings us into the present. When you put your
attention on each breath, you guarantee a shift toward optimal mental
and physical health. It is a fact of nature. When we take a break, we
give our genie a break. We come back from the break with the clarity
of mind to refresh our entire life process. After all, the mind can be our
worst enemy, or our best friend, in a very real and powerful sense.

So far, what we have been talking about is focused breathing
with your everyday, ordinary breath. But breathing feels different in
different moments. There is the sitting-down-after-exertion breath, a
standing breath, and a reclining breath. However, you can ride each
of these types of breath with intention and awareness. Not to do so
merely compounds our naturally challenging lives and pulls our focus
away from our core life energy. It locks us into a stress wish, which
only creates a snowball of asphyxiation that keeps our cells from
breathing. Next time you find yourself on a stress ride, take a breath
ride. Your body and teen genie will be glad you did.

## Constant Breathing

Remember the constant breath I mentioned earlier? It is the breath
that moves you through your day. Become more conscious of it, and
your life will be richer and fuller as a result. It's important to remember,
however, that consciousness isn't about thinking. It's about feeling.

There is a subtle but important difference between experiencing
a feeling and thinking about a feeling. The object here is not to
*think* about how your body feels, but to *simply* feel it. *Allow* the
experience. As soon as you think, "Am I doing this right?" or "I have
to be conscious of my breathing," you have entered the constricted
mental space that you are trying to leave behind. If such thoughts
arise, acknowledge them and return your focus to the feeling of
rhythmic breathing. This awareness, which I call, "being in the body,"
is important to a successful breathing practice, in that it facilitates

consciously noting the feedback your body provides. Being aware of what you feel as you breathe can take you to unlimited possibilities. Besides, we think too much anyway.

## The Breathing Myth

Many people think that conscious breathing is something that is New Age, or they think it's a difficult practice exclusive to gurus or followers of Eastern yoga and meditation that is out of reach for most of us. I say that, while you may have a different lifestyle than Guru Ji or a yogi, we all breathe the same air. It is the one thing that everyone shares. You certainly do not need to be a guru to grasp the essential and immediate importance of having our 30 trillion cells enjoy a healthy supply of vital oxygen! No matter who you are or where you live, your body is already wired, via the nervous and muscular systems, to breathe slowly and fully. Remember, babies are excellent breathers, and at one time we were all babies. Conscious, slow breathing is a built-in means for all of us to access our inner youth of conscious awareness.

For me, breathing is so significant because, after practicing rhythmic breathing for one week, my life changed—my stutter went away. And it never returned. It had been my wheelchair, and when I got out of it, I never went back. As a clinician, instead of giving my patients medication, I show them how to meditate on breath. Breathing is wonderful because, unlike medication, you do not need to buy it or receive it. You already possess it—or rather, it possesses you. It is there with you always, bringing with it vital oxygenation for your entire being. Breathing is a direct connection to what life is all about. If you were to ask, "What is the self?" I would have to say, "It's that energy that breathes my life."

## Rhythmic Breathing

When you are rhythmically breathing, you experience a visual sense of your body doing it for you. Any time you think about breathing, you stifle your breath. This especially applies to rhythmic breathing. Your body already knows how to breathe rhythmically, just like it knows how to walk across the room. You don't have think about it; you just let your body do its thing and it will get you there.

Remember, it is your muscles that breathe you. When you feel your abdominal, back, and diaphragm muscles contract and expand with rhythm, they naturally want to continue breathing that way. One more time—the key is *not* to think about it.

### The Story of the Young Sailor

After hearing about the old Polynesian sailor who navigated the ocean without so much as a compass, a young American sailor arranged to meet him for an apprenticeship in Hawaii. The younger sailor wanted so much to learn the old ways and to navigate via the wind, the swell, the sun, the moon, and the entire Milky Way. Expecting to spend at least a year studying with the old sailor, he was surprised to learn this ancient form of navigation in one lesson.

The two of them met on a boulder overlooking the ocean. The old sailor told the young sailor, "Close your eyes and see Australia and now feel it as if you are already there."

The young sailor closed his eyes and began to visualize the continent.

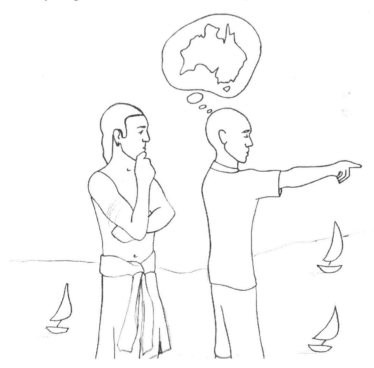

"Now point to it," the older sailor said.

When the young man motioned in the direction of Australia, the older sailor said, "The lesson is complete. You have learned the ancient ways!"

This story most readily applies to rhythmic breathing: First, you see it, then you feel it, and then, like magic, it appears the first time you internally observe and feel your breath's rhythm.

## Breath-breathing Dragons

Since breath is the most immediate life energy, it plays a vital role in maintaining good health.

Health experts say that we are what we eat. We are also what we drink and, most importantly, what we breathe—and how we breathe it. Human beings can live without food for four weeks, without water for four days, but without air for only four minutes. On any given day, we eat three meals and maybe snack in between. But during that same day, as mentioned earlier, approximately 23,000 cycles of respiration pass through each of us.

When we breathe through our noses, the air is cleaned and regulated to the body's proper humidity and temperature before it enters the lungs.

When the blood passes through the lungs, the oxygen is magnetized to red blood cells and it then begins its epic journey through thousands of miles of channels in the body, oxygenating the body's cells along the way. When the oxygen molecule arrives at the cell, its membrane opens and the inner cellular world gladly receives the oxygen, bringing with it a breath of fresh air. The cell heats the oxygen slightly to bring it to just the right temperature, takes what it needs, and sends it on its way again back through the membrane, into the blood, and then back into the atmosphere. By this time, the air in your body is warm and includes a mix of everything the cells want to send back into the atmosphere. We are like breath-breathing dragons, taking in the cool atmosphere, bringing it to a simmer, and then blowing out the warmth of the inner cellular atmosphere.

Deep, rhythmic breathing is not just healthy, it is essential for each and every cell. The cells love it, and in return, they maintain an awesome life vibration. Being aware of your breath is the committed and cherished practice of receiving rather than taking. This gently reassures us that the pulse of life breathes on.

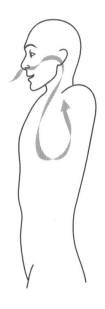
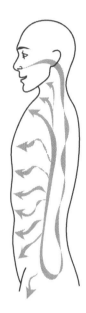

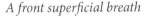

*A front superficial breath*          *A deep back breath*

## Relearning the Full Breath

When most people think of a full breath, they think of the chest and upper abdomen expanding. This breath is actually a stress reflex designed to suck in a lot of air quickly and get it out. However, when we direct the air down along the inner side of the spinal column, it engages the full range of breathing muscles that draw the breath deep into the lungs. The entire torso expands, moving the joints and organs, expanding the rib cage out in all directions. Imagine that you are breathing from the back of your body to the front rather than from the front to the back.

When you practice full back breathing regularly, it will eventually become part of your everyday breathing, making your regular breath stronger, smoother, and more rhythmic. So as you move through your day, periodically take three to four conscious, slow, deep back breaths. Feel the breath going down your backside, moving your base, expanding into your frontal body, opening up your abdomen, and going upward into your chest. Breathe deep into your backside and then feel it expand your front torso upward. Taking three or four deep breaths whenever you can remember to do it will condition your regular breathing to be richer and fuller. It will become your body's regular way of breathing, thus providing for a calmer nervous system and less stress. Try it! This form of breathing employs your parasympathetic nervous system, which reduces your stress levels.

### Getting Reacquainted with Regular Breathing

> *"The warrior who lives on the outside is not afraid of dying.*
> *The warrior who lives on the inside is not afraid of living."*
>
> – Lao Tzu

All of the practices in this book are designed to support and enhance your regular breath. Compare breathing practice to working out—with breathing, you're working in. People regularly put aside time to work out, but we don't always take quiet time to explore the feeling of our breath and to hone in on how amazing it feels to breathe deeply and slowly. The early morning before the day begins is a great time to practice conscious breathing.

Simply being conscious of your breath as it flows in and out of you is the first step in developing a healthy breathing pattern. Focusing on your regular breath gives you an inner awareness of where your body is internally. The body follows the breath, so if your breath is quick and erratic, your metabolism will also be quick and erratic. When your breath is smooth and rhythmic, your metabolism flows more smoothly and rhythmically. By drawing attention to your everyday breath, you are paying attention to nature's life-sustaining atmosphere flowing in and out of you. You are also taking a break from random mental chatter.

## EXERCISE: *Full Breaths*

Now let us try a few full body breaths. Lie down and place one hand on your abdomen. Place the other hand wherever it feels good. (My personal favorite is behind the base of the skull, as this region has acupuncture points for treating mental and emotional conditions). Take a deep, unforced inhale. Now, notice how the breath feels as you listen to the sound of the faintest whisper of air as it flows through your nose and opens up your face. Follow the next inhale down along your spine to its base where it expands into your lower torso. Then follow it as it flows to the front of your body and upward into your chest.

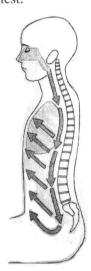

Next, feel the massaging breath exerting pressure on your internal organs and spinal muscles. Be open to these sensations and enjoy this connection. Pay attention to the signals your body sends to let you know how far down your breath has reached. Is your pelvis expanding? What about your lower abdomen and rib cage? Is the hand on your abdomen rising with your breath?

Bring your awareness even deeper by pausing for a moment before you gently exhale. Continue to direct your feelings and awareness into your breath. Do not criticize yourself if you have trouble feeling your belly expand—just feel your breath and chaaa!

### *Nose Power*

According to Honolulu orthodontist and creator of the Nose Breathe Mouthpiece, Dr. Steven K. Sue, nose breathing improves coordination, increases stamina and endurance, prevents over-straining, decreases mucous production, reduces the pulse rate, places less stress on the heart, improves oxygenation of the blood, and reduces snoring. He has stated his surprise at the "magnitude of health issues associated with incorrect breathing," and believes it has affected every facet of our society.

Take a relaxed breath through your nose, and then take one through your mouth. The nose breath feels as if it is flowing through your face, opening up your entire head as it regulates the air before it enters your lungs. Mouth breathing, on the other hand, can feel like gulping down air and has been known to increase stress levels.

Nose breathing prepares the air before it enters the lungs by regulating temperature and humidity, correcting and balancing each breath. The fine nasal hairs and a layer of sticky mucus membrane serve as a filter to capture airborne particles such as dust, allergens, and even bacteria that enter through the nasal passages. As air flows through the nose, it swirls around, passing by the body's temperature and humidity controlling centers. The air then enters the three sinus cavities called turbinate bones that resemble elongated seashells. On the inside of these seashell-like cavities are turbine-shaped designs, thus the name turbinate bones. They aerodynamically swirl the air along curved walls designed to promote air flow across the maximum surface area. Along the way, the air collects moisture to achieve the proper humidity of 98 percent water saturation. The air is also regulated to the body's temperature before it enters the lungs (somewhere between 32–34° or 89–93°F). If these turbinating mechanisms malfunctioned or stopped working, the body's inner furnace would quickly cool down.

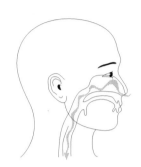

Breathing naturally through your nostrils serves your entire body. As each breath moves through your nasal pathways, it opens up and relaxes your entire facial area, giving a treat to the sensory organs located there. Breathing through your mouth bypasses this vital system, so it's important to breathe nasally whenever possible.

If you would like to try enhancing your nasal breathing, begin practicing in short spans of time. You might also practice nasal breathing with your mouth gently taped shut during normal activities like walking around the house, washing the dishes—performing your daily routine. Start gently with the taping of the mouth, slowly increasing the amount of time you spend this way, and soon you will improve and open up your nasal airways to healthy breathing. Gradually your body will acclimate to it, producing a much healthier nasal capacity. And soon, you won't need the tape as a reminder!

## EXERCISE: *Opening Your Nasal Pathways*

Most of us have no problem breathing through our noses, but when you are congested you may need to make more of an effort. You can use your fingers or thumbs to help you open up your nasal pathways. Try placing your thumbs or middle fingers to the sides of both nostrils. Press both sides until you feel a degree of discomfort. Then press and stretch the nostrils toward your ears, along the top edge of your cheekbones.

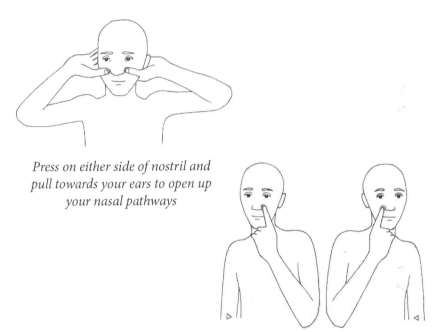

*Press on either side of nostril and pull towards your ears to open up your nasal pathways*

*As above but using one finger*

    When you do this, you are pressing into an acupuncture point that is used to treat nasal congestion. Most people are tender on this pressure point, so when you feel tenderness there, press into it and stretch the nostrils outward. Pressing these points and stretching toward your ears opens up your nasal capacity and provides relief from congestion.

## Optimal Breathing

We all have different body types. Therefore, there is no absolute right way for everyone to breathe. There is, however, an optimal way for you, individually, to breathe. In order to find your optimal breathing, you must explore the practice of diaphragmatic breathing.

### *The Muscle that Breathes You*

The thoracic diaphragm muscle is truly amazing and is responsible for some 75 percent of healthy respiratory function—this is the muscle that breathes you. Shaped somewhat like an umbrella traversing the mid-torso, separating the upper torso from the lower, it connects to the ribs and breastbone. It fans upward to connect to the heart and lungs by way of string-like tissue called fascia. The diaphragm and the lower abdominal muscles are the main players in full, healthy respiration.

When we inhale, the diaphragm muscle contracts and creates a concave, downward shape. This action opens up space in the lungs, creating a vacuum effect that is quickly filled with air. The diaphragmatic action during inhalation presses downward into the belly of the abdomen, performing an inner massage that moves the organs and inner body parts. The diaphragm is attached to the heart— each inhalation gently pulls on the heart, which in turn facilitates healthier cardiac function.

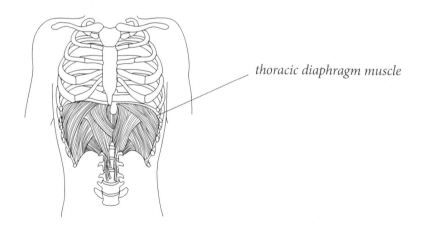

*thoracic diaphragm muscle*

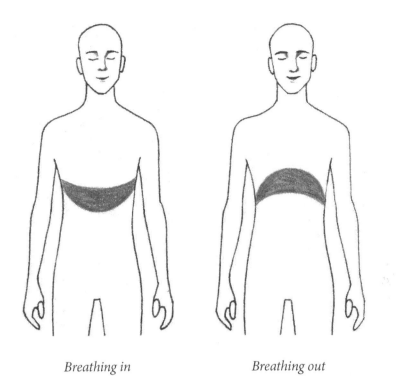

*Breathing in*                    *Breathing out*

The diaphragm muscle extends downward and has a tail that attaches to the lower back so when you breathe into its base, it contracts and expands, serving as a lubricant to the muscles, joints, and organs of the lower body. A full diaphragmatic inhalation will also draw the air deeper into the lungs where there is more blood supply to the alveoli (also known as air sacks). Think of alveoli as suction pads that suck in oxygen and blow out carbon dioxide. The upper part of the lungs does not have such a rich supply of capillaries to the alveoli. That means that when you breathe superficially, you are not receiving a healthy exchange of oxygen to carbon dioxide ($CO_2$).

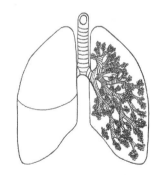

*When you breathe from your deep muscles, you utilize the full capacity of your lungs.*

When the diaphragm muscle relaxes, it puts pressure on the lungs to exude its contents. Because these full exhalations expel the heavier body waste in the lower parts of the lungs, this is another way the body purifies itself.

Other muscles that play supporting roles in breathing include the abdominal and back muscles, the throat and pelvic diaphragm muscles, the intercostal muscles, the muscles on the sides of the neck, and the upper chest muscles. It is important to remember that all of these muscles work together to ensure that we maintain the correct quotas of oxygen and $CO_2$ in our bodies.

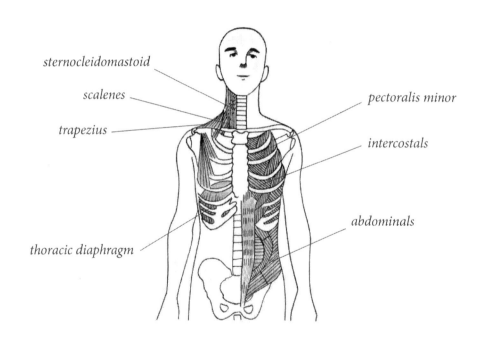

Stress-affected breathing disengages the thoracic diaphragm and lower muscles, then delegates the work to the upper chest and neck muscles. The upper chest and neck muscles are not strong lower muscles. They are not designed for long-term breathing. They tire, tighten up, and can even cause pain. This may lead to the tendency to hyperventilate, as I will discuss later in Chapter 5: Hyperventilation. Subsequently, a type of "on-and-off" breathing develops in which you hold your breath, especially during stress, and then you begin sucking in large amounts of air to compensate. When you breathe primarily into your upper chest, you do not benefit from receiving a healthy air supply and internal organ massage. Deep, diaphragmatic breathing is our natural design. To breathe well is the most awesome thing you can do for yourself. So breathe slowly and deeply!

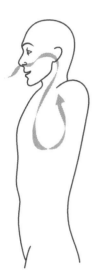
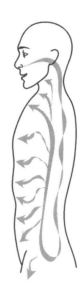

*Shallow front breath*    *Deep back breath*

### *Breathing into Your Pyramid*

Many people, especially when they are stressed, live in what I call an upside-down pyramid breath. The upside-down pyramid breath is a very common form of stressful breathing. It elevates the shoulders and the breathing is shallow and occurs mainly in the upper lungs. The next time you catch yourself in an upside-down pyramid, imagine the pyramid in your mind, turn it right side up, and breathe into its base—into your thoracic diaphragm and lower lungs. The body responds by taking a deep, slow breath, filling up the base of the pyramid, using your breathing muscles and lungs to the fullest. Continue to visualize your breath as an upright pyramid so when you breathe in, you fill the base of your pyramid, thus utilizing your full lung capacity.

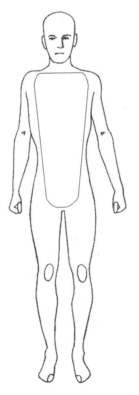 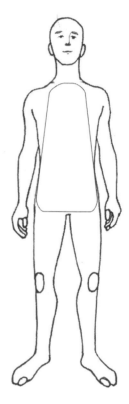

*The upside down superficial stressful pyramid breath*

*The right side up deep pyramid breath*

This method of breathing is a highly effective way to reverse the instinct to freeze up so you can regulate your breath. It sets your body in a new direction that moves you while it oxygenates your core. When stress takes hold, release it by breathing deeply into it. This will create healthy patterns of breathing in your body, and it will keep you from responding to stress by suspending your vital breath, which only causes the overreaction of breathing quickly and sucking in air.

You cannot stop breathing. However, the choice is yours as to whether you breathe rhythmically and consciously throughout the day or erratically without awareness. Personally, I like to smell and listen to my breath. I can even taste it. With every breath of fresh air you breathe, remember to go slowly and deeply and feel the chaaa!

## EXERCISE: *Diaphragmatic Strengthening by Resistance*

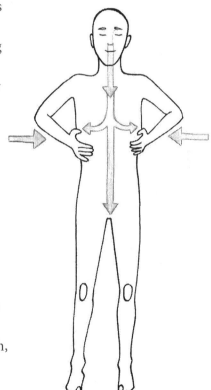

This exercise is like doing pushups for the muscles that breathe you. You can perform it either standing or lying down. Place both hands around the front and sides of your rib cage with your fingers facing forward and, as you take a deep breath, exert pressure with your hands to resist the expansion of your lungs. Your emphasis should be on resistance upon your inhalation, specifically. This pushes the diaphragm muscle downward, massaging the organs, and moving the lower body, thus challenging and strengthening the diaphragm muscle.

Do this for five cycles of breath, resting for 30 seconds in between. Then repeat it another five times.

Breathe slowly and remember to resist the inhalation. When you have completed this diaphragmatic breathing practice, you will notice a free, expansive breath in your body and an open sense of breathing a smoother, fuller breath.

Try taking deep diaphragmatic back breaths three or four times while sitting at the computer or at a red light in traffic. Notice the deep breath go down the back side of your body then toward the front, expanding your whole frontal torso, all the way up to your head and the neck.

### EXERCISE: *Body-Focused Isolated Breathing*

One of the most powerful ways to use breath as a tool for healing is to determine the internal status of your body. If you are like many people, you need that status report. Anatomically focused breathing, or isolated breathing, requires breathing into your body parts. It may be a muscle, a joint, an internal organ, or any body part that is calling for your attention. Patients of mine who have tried this technique have reported not only relief from the pain, but also a genuine healing of their underlying condition.

You can do this in any position, as long as you are comfortable and free of any restrictions (like tight clothing). Start with a minute or so of rhythmic breathing. Pay specific attention to any area of your body where you are carrying tension, strain, or pain. Allow your mind to drift into that area, and then follow it with your breath. Now, without forcing or grabbing, ease a deep, slow breath right into the painful area. Fill the tense or sore spot with breath. On your exhalation, let the tension go as you exhale it away and chaaa into a state of peaceful awareness.

Within minutes of this isolated, slow breathing, you will dramatically improve the flow of energy to the constricted or painful area and experience a sense of relief. For example, to relieve tension in your lower back, take a slow deep breath from your diaphragm and lower breathing muscles, and direct your breath down into your lower back. Feel the muscles and joints move as you breathe. You can also use this form of breathing in any first-aid situation. Increasing energy flow to the affected area will significantly improve your chances of a speedy recovery.

One of the greatest aspects of conscious breathing is that it provides a simple and immediate avenue of positive response to almost any situation. When stress causes you to trigger your internal panic button, you can choose breath to guide you to an alternative way of observing the situation rather than reacting to it. When we choose breath over panic, we no longer need to spend life's energy overreacting to the stories we create in our minds after a panic moment has passed. When you feel stuck in something or don't know what to do, the best thing is to breathe consciously, slowly, and deeply. When you focus on your breath, it takes you out of your head, allowing you to access a deep body intelligence so that no matter what you face, your responses become more effective.

If you apply the process of conscious breathing into your everyday life, even for five minutes three times a day, you can make a big difference in your health.

### EXERCISE: *The Rub and Cup Eye Saver*
This practice is especially good for those of us who stare at screens.

If you wear contact lenses, remove them before you begin. Rub the palms of your hands together until you generate some heat in them. Cup your hands and place one hand over each eye and breathe deeply. Inhale and feel the warm energy from your hands enter your eyes. In your mind's eye, visualize your exhalation going out through your hands. You may feel a tingling sensation all around your eyes. After two breath cycles, rub your hands together again and repeat. Just chaaa. This simple exercise helps calms the nervous system, clear the eyes, and release the surrounding muscle tension. Do this often during screen time.

*"A person who is a master in the art of living makes little distinction between their work and their play, their labor and their leisure, their mind and their body, their education and their recreation, their love and religion. They hardly know which is which and simply pursue their vision of excellence and grace in whatever they do, leaving others to decide whether they are working or playing. To them they are always doing both."*

– Lawrence Pearsall Jacks

## Breathing Away Acute Anxiety

A patient of mine named Jack was an aspiring actor looking for his big break. The problem, he said, was that every time he went to an audition, he tensed up and his face began to twitch with a nervous tic. When casting directors saw his handsome face twitching, they quickly crossed his name off their callback lists. I felt great compassion for him because his tic reminded me of my stammer. The doctors he had seen recommended a typical solution for his problem—a muscle relaxant. I watched him closely as he described his condition and my first observation was that his breathing was high up in his chest, which caused his neck and facial muscles to tense. This, in turn, made his whole body tighten up. Instead of prescribing a pill, I taught him the same breathing technique that helped me release my stutter some decades ago.

The results changed his life. "When I softly bend my knees and direct four or five slow, non-forced breaths right into the place where the nervous feeling is—often found in my gut—I then resume observing the flow of being breathed deeply," he told me, "I was amazed at how quickly my body readjusted itself." He practiced this technique often, and, as a result, it became second nature. He repeated it intensely before his auditions in order to relax. I don't think about the symptoms anymore because they're gone."

It was obvious to me that while some doctors wanted to treat him with drugs, Jack could treat himself with what he really needed—oxygen and the relaxation that comes with having enough full breath.

When our breath is freely flowing, we can feel a sense of being open from the inside out. When we breathe, there is an expansion and contraction like a wave that travels through us, moving our muscles and bones. Even our skin expands. Indeed, there is an energy field that extends out in all directions; you can feel it in the peripheral parts of your body. When you practice breathing, it is important to breathe into your whole body and feel the rhythmic wave of breath move through you.

## EXERCISE: *Bad Mood Busting Breath*

Did you know that the physiological act of smiling increases the level of "happy" chemicals in your brain? It's true—the actual muscles involved in smiling directly affect your brain chemistry. A frown has the opposite effect. When we suffer from being in a bad mood, our natural tendency is to frown, but this only makes the bad mood worse. So at the risk of sounding goofy—turn that frown upside down and smile! (This exercise works even if you mimic a smile.)

This practice is easy: Stand, sit, or lie down comfortably. Smile as you breathe and enjoy the process.

## EXERCISE: *Smiling at Someone Beautiful*

Have you ever noticed that it feels good when you smile at someone (even a stranger) and you receive a smile back? So try smiling more—even at strangers.

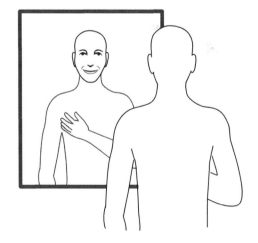

Now try this. It may seem silly, but try looking into a mirror while smiling. As you do this, realize that you are smiling at someone beautiful, and see that beautiful person smiling back.

**EXERCISE:** *A Variation on Smiling at Someone Beautiful*

Do the above exercise and go from smiling to laughing, even if you have to fake it a little at first. And then let the laugh go—all the way into a deep belly laugh. Feel the laughter from every cell in your body.

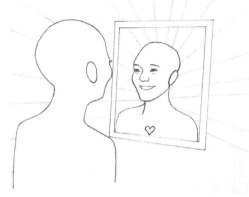

When you feel that overall laughter, your body is laughing with you. It is not that you are laughing *at* yourself, although that is fine too, but rather, you're laughing because you are happy. Who better to laugh with than yourself? This feeling is naturally blissful. A full breath and a great laugh changes our moods, as well as the thoughts we think about each other and ourselves.

**EXERCISE:** *Another Great Mood Enhancer*

When I first graduated from acupuncture school in Sydney in 1975, I volunteered my services in a heroin withdrawal clinic.

During acupuncture with patients at the clinic, I realized how effective acupuncture treatment can be on a person who is going through cold-turkey heroin withdrawal. After only 20 minutes of needling and sending an electrical current through the needle, the patient's nervous system calms down dramatically.

You can create a similar effect by lying down and placing your right hand at the base of your skull where there are mind-calming acupressure points, and then placing your left hand on a traditional acupuncture point called the dan tien, located just below the belly button. In martial arts practices, this point is considered the center. Based on traditional acupuncture, this area revitalizes the body's vital energy, inviting longevity. By placing your right hand on the base of your skull and your left hand on the dan tien, you are connecting to your central nervous system and your base energetic system.

*When you touch the back of your head you are connecting to potent acupuncture points designed to soothe the nervous system.*

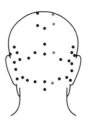

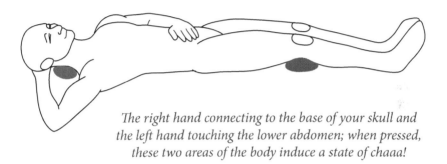

*The right hand connecting to the base of your skull and the left hand touching the lower abdomen; when pressed, these two areas of the body induce a state of chaaa!*

Additionally, by laying your hands on these powerful energy points, you will become aware of the transmission of energy between your hands and the back of your head. The exchange of this energy has a soothing effect on your entire nervous system. While you may not be going through heroin withdrawal, all of us are going through something. No matter what that is, you will still feel the benefits of allowing this exchange of energy to take place as you chaaa yourself into awareness.

I have already highlighted the importance of feeling rather than thinking. Now let us take it a step further. As your hands feel your body, become aware of your body feeling your hands. Be receptive to the exchange of energy from your hands to your body and from your body to your hands. To become more aware, feel the energy connection between the left hand you placed on the back of your head and your right hand, just below your belly button. Stay with that feeling as your awareness drifts into a complete body energy connection.

From here, you can feel essential base energy, which gives you a sense of being grounded. As you lie in this state, always remember to check in on the rhythm of your breath. The secret is not to think about it but rather to see and feel the breath reach a natural rhythm.

Inhale slowly down into your lower back and pelvis, then follow your breath up into your solar plexus, feeling it as it lifts your chest and ascends upward through your neck, into your head, and fills up your entire being. As you exhale, concentrate on the back of your head as you slowly let go from a deep exhalation. Take 10 breaths like this, and then resume regular breathing into your whole body—keep smiling!

## EXERCISE: *Evening Breath*

In the morning when I wake, it is as if I am taking off like an airplane into my day. The evening time is when I come in to land. But both morning and evening are conducive to rest and to conscious breath awareness. And as such, even if your body follows a different rhythm, you can benefit from this practice.

If you are one of those people who say a prayer before sleep, you may want to include a moment of focused breathing in your practice. Before going to sleep, it is a good idea to take some time to consciously breathe.

You may find that your mind refuses to turn off when you try to go to sleep at night. You may tell yourself, "Think happy thoughts so you can relax." This may work sometimes, but certainly not always.

If there are any daytime issues lingering in your body, acknowledge them, feel them, and direct 10 rhythmic breaths into those feelings. After that, resume natural rhythmic breathing. This is an effective way to air out lingering tensions from the day—and it also clears the way for a restful, deep sleep. You will awaken in the morning feeling rested, energetic, and once again ready to joyfully invite in the morning breath.

Sleep is an unconscious state. Good intentions work wonders here. In other words, direct your intentions toward a deep, restful, comfortable sleep. Remember that, even in sleep, your intention is to breathe rhythmically as you enjoy deep unconsciousness.

**EXERCISE:** *Good Morning Breath*

While filming *Power Healing*, my video about breath work, Ringo Starr said, "When I first wake up in the morning, my mind is like a minefield. And through meditation, prayer, and breathing, the mines are defused." If your experience is anything like his, you'll gain a great deal from making this practice a habit.

The early morning before you get out of bed to begin the day is a great time to focus on your breath. Personally, I turn my attention to my breath and simply observe the flow in and out. Periodically, it feels good to stretch and then lie still again in a comfortable position and continue to enjoy the awareness of my breath. Starting your day with conscious breathing will carry through into the rest of your daytime breathing, giving it more depth and awareness.

## Checking In

Remember to check in with your breath throughout the day. Do not judge yourself based on how tense you may be or whether you are holding stressful thoughts. Simply bring awareness to your body and allow yourself to breathe. Soon you will calm your mind and enter the energy within your breath. This energy is where we get to know our true selves, the selves beyond our thoughts. It is also a place where healing and regeneration occur. Remember that breathing is free and you can practice it wherever you are! Simply engaging in five deep breaths five times a day will strengthen the muscles that breathe you, allowing for fuller, richer regular breath.

# CHAPTER FIVE

# *Breath Holders and Hyperventilation*

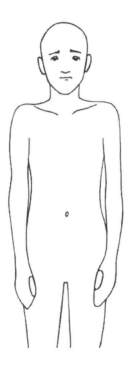

## Breath Holders

During the course of any given day, many of us habitually hold our breath. We become so concentrated on a thought or external nuances that we literally go unconscious. At a sporting event, when our team is losing or about to score, we stop breathing. At the workplace when we're being reprimanded, or when we are about to make a presentation, we can freeze. There is a sigh of relief when the tension is resolved and the drama, real or imagined, fades. By far, the most common breath stranglers always lurking close by are stressful thoughts. Memories and confrontations, real or otherwise, can occupy the space reserved for calm, focused breath.

The reality is that when we are holding our breath, we are impaired. And holding your breath when you're stressed is like actively pushing your own panic button. In those moments, you do, in fact, lose your breath. Your senses are compromised, your awareness is depleted, and in chronic cases, your organs and internal pathways can be adversely affected. Holding your breath is like prematurely throwing in the towel on life—at least for a few moments.

Conversely, it is an act of utmost self-respect, restoration, and kindness to slowly ride your breath for all it is worth. Remember that its worth is immeasurable. Breathing is simple, natural, and exists to be optimized. No pill, tool, or remedy can replace it or even come close. The choice is yours—take a leap, and, instead of holding your breath during a stressful moment, choose conscious, slow breathing.

When you cannot run and are too afraid to fight, try taking a deep, slow back breath all the way into your pelvis. Remember to breathe through your nose. This will keep you from falling into the habit of freezing and then hyperventilating. When you forget to breathe, whatever the reason, the nervous system switches on the fight, flight, or freeze reflex and it's easy to become anxious, irritable, and nervous. Hyperventilation often comes with these feelings, and that is a condition we must avoid. But when you handle stress by consciously taking slow, deep breaths, you alter the stress response pattern that causes you to press your panic button. This slow, focused breath produces an opening within you and gives you a new and wider perspective on yourself and the world around you. Allow your breath to take you out of your head and into a deeper mind-body intelligence.

## Hyperventilation

Hyperventilation, though it is a *common* reaction to stress, is not a *good* reaction to stress. In fact, hyperventilating during times of stress causes a host of physiological changes and, as a result, increases your stress. Hyperventilation is public enemy number one.

## Physiological Results of Hyperventilation

Hyperventilation often begins with the tendency to hold one's breath under duress. The result is that your blood becomes starved of oxygen, leading the nervous system to press the panic button. It overreacts and tells the respiratory center in the brain to speed up your breathing. Then you take in deep, rapid breaths, or you begin to hurry your breathing, sucking in shallow amounts of air through your mouth. Your blood then goes from being oxygen-starved to being oxygen-rich, creating an imbalance in the blood gases. The carbon dioxide cannot keep up with the oxygen that you created through your accelerated breathing, and this leads to a host of physiological changes, including constricting the blood flow to your brain, kidneys, and intestines. Hyperventilation can also cause lightheadedness and, in severe cases, convulsions and unconsciousness.

We all know the importance of oxygen, but most people are unaware of the importance of carbon dioxide. Perhaps this is because $CO_2$ is a metabolic waste product, the body breathes it out, so it is not typically regarded as an essential respiratory molecule. $CO_2$, however, is vital because it regulates blood pH and thus regulates the effective availability of oxygen to the cells.

When you breathe too quickly, there is a sudden infusion of oxygen in your blood. As I mentioned earlier, the carbon dioxide cannot keep up with the high levels of oxygen. When the blood becomes too deficient in $CO_2$, the blood pH rises or becomes more alkaline. Under ideal pH levels, oxygen is loosely bonded to hemoglobin in the red blood cell, allowing the oxygen molecule to be easily released into oxygen-deprived tissues. Excessively alkaline blood conditions (those that are higher than 7.35 pH) cause the bond between the hemoglobin and oxygen to strengthen, so the oxygen is less likely to be released into the cells where it's needed.

The hemoglobin inside the red blood cell becomes saturated with oxygen, while the surrounding tissues become starved of oxygen. This acts as a trigger for the pituitary gland to increase your respiratory rate, which only exacerbates the problem—you hyperventilate more.

In Dr. Robert Fried's book, *The Breath Connection*, he cites several studies that demonstrate a host of mental, stress-related, psychological, and physiological adverse changes that follow hyperventilation. Dr. Fried recognizes hyperventilation as one of the most underdiagnosed health conditions in society.

The effects of low carbon dioxide are well documented in medical books. Take, for example, these excerpts from a 1978 *Journal of the American Medical Association* study on hyperventilation:

Hyperventilation syndrome is a common, often disabling and frequently inadequately treated clinical problem. Indeed, many patients with this affliction wander from one physician to another either vainly undergoing increasingly complex diagnostic procedures or being dismissed as anxious or neurotic.

The study includes a table of symptoms believed to be related to hyperventilation:

Fatigue, exhaustion, heart palpitations, rapid pulse, dizziness, lightheadedness, disturbances of consciousness or vision, numbness and tingling in the limbs, shortness of breath, yawning, chest pain, feeling of a lump in the throat, stomach pain, involuntary contraction of muscles, cramps and tremors, stiffness, anxiety, insomnia and nightmares, impairment of concentration and memory.

Some authorities believe that bad breathing habits may be primarily responsible for the hyperventilation syndrome and that anxiety is secondary.

As far back as 1559, Dulaurens noted, "Melancholoke folke are commonly given to sigh, because the mind being possessed with great varietie and store of foolish apparitions doth not remember or suffer the parite [parity] to be at leisure to breathe according to the necessitie of nature." This ancient passage serves to remind us that healthy breathing is not a New Age idea.

Traditional Chinese doctors have understood for thousands of years that when a person's breathing is healthy, the whole body is healthy.

## When Your Breath is Fast and Erratic, Slow It Down

The best cure for hyperventilation, without a doubt, is simple, slow, rhythmic breathing. When you are rhythmically breathing, you experience a visual sense of your body doing it for you. (Hyperventilation, on the other hand, is quite a gasping, chest-heaving effort.)

## Inducing Hyperventilation

My good friend and neighbor, Jonny, shared his experience with me. He described what happened to him when his girlfriend offered him a gift. Jonny thought he was going to receive a massage, but instead it was something quite different. His girlfriend told him, "You are going to be rebirthed."

The practitioner who conducted the treatment asked Jonny to lie down on his back and relax. In this method of rebirthing, the person receiving it takes quick, superficial breaths through the mouth while lying still, which alters the person's state of mind and body. She then instructed him to take quick, short breaths though his mouth. After five minutes of quick breathing through his mouth, Jonny's fingers, legs, and arms felt cold, numb, and tingly. As he continued to breathe through his mouth, his mouth and face became stiff—indeed his whole body stiffened. After 25 minutes, Jonny was in a fetal position, his round-shaped mouth was frozen, and he could not open or close it. Once the half-hour practice was finally complete, Jonny remained stuck in a fetal position. The practitioner told Jonny that he would be OK—his reaction was common. "It took me a half an hour before I began break out of the fetal position and be able to move again." Jonny described his experience as traumatizing and has no desire to try rebirthing again.

## The Great Misconception

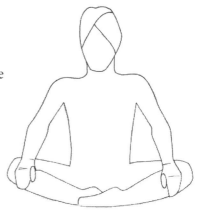

Too much of a good thing can be a bad thing. This applies to excessive eating, drinking, *and* breathing. Some forms of yoga and meditation—and rebirthing—require deep, rapid breathing for long periods while sitting or lying still. I would like to make a precautionary observation about rapid breathing practices: When we breathe deeply and rapidly while in a physically passive (non-aerobic) state, we participate in a form of hyperventilation. We gulp large volumes of oxygen and then lose carbon dioxide faster than the body's tissues can absorb it. Remember that, under ideal circumstances, the blood's pH is around 7.35 (slightly alkaline). When the cells become deficient in $CO_2$, the blood pH rises or becomes more alkaline. This impairs the transport of oxygen to the brain, heart, kidneys, and other organs.

Some still regard rapid, deep breathing or "sucking in" air while you're in a passive state as a healthy practice. Perhaps they believe the theory that more is better applies here. In reality, however, when it comes to rapid, deep breathing, less is better. We should practice a small amount of this type of breathing to stimulate circulation, and then *return* to regular breathing.

To reiterate, the body is not designed to take in large volumes of air while it is physically inactive. This excessive form of breathing is hyperventilating and should be done only in small durations of no more than one minute at a time. If you practice this form of breathing, it is important for you to stretch or shake before, during, and after each practice.

Again let us also remind ourselves who eventually won the race between the tortoise and the hair. In the real animal world, faster-breathing animals actually do live shorter lives. Remember that we too are designed to breathe slowly and rhythmically. It is simple, slow, rhythmic breathing that is our inner power, sustaining us for a long life.

**EXERCISE:** *Airing Out Painful Issues*

When we are holding on to a painful issue, whether it is emotional, mental, or physical, our first tendency is to either deny it or turn to a health care professional to help us ameliorate the symptoms the issue is causing. Though both of these coping mechanisms might work for a short period of time, neither do the work of moving us through the painful issue. When we breathe into that painful issue instead, we no longer deny it— we do, in fact, "air it out." By breathing into an issue, we can stop analyzing it and simply breathe into it to release and move the painful energy. When something moves, it can no longer be stuck.

Here's how you can practice airing out. Every time an issue appears in your life, find out where you can feel it in your body. Feelings and memories are anatomically located somewhere in all of us. The great thing about being in the moment and internally conscious is that we can see where these feelings are located in our bodies.

To begin this exercise, lie down in a chaaa state and practice one or two full body breaths. As you do, scan your body slowly, starting with your toes, feeling for any pain, constriction, or blockages. They may be in more than one location. The back of the neck, the lower back, the gut, the solar plexus and the chest are places where feelings often show up in the body. Once you locate where the issue is stuck, start by practicing slow, conscious, directed breathing right into the center of it—feel it, try to see it, and imagine it opening.

Sometimes our painful issues are directed at others and can become stuck in our psyches, turning into grudges. Bad feelings or bad memories all serve to constrict and deplete our life energy. Any time you feel this happening, or when you are in any stressful moment, find it in your body and complete a cycle of 10 breaths directed into the center of the feeling. By so doing, you begin the process of releasing your inner fixations and letting go of the past. You can apply this practice to anything—anger, resentment, sadness, despair, anguish, loss, grief, or physical pain.

As you air out your old issues, it is also profoundly helpful to adopt an attitude of forgiveness. You may not be able to forget, but forgiving and breathing into an issue is a powerful healing choice— and it provides an awesome opportunity for you to move on.

When we are unable to let something go to the extent that it becomes stuck in our bodies as pain or discomfort of any kind, or even as hyperventilation, it is usually because we have not moved out of the realm of thinking about the issue. It is so easy to fall into the trap of thinking rather than feeling. This principle especially applies when you are breathing into your inner mental and emotional fixations. You may realize that you are breathing into your thoughts on the issues or even into a mental picture of it. But you will enjoy sustainable improvement when you can differentiate between thinking and feeling, and indeed, when you can direct your breathing into the emotional or physical location of the problem, rather than into the image or words you apply to it.

# CHAPTER SIX
## *Alignment*

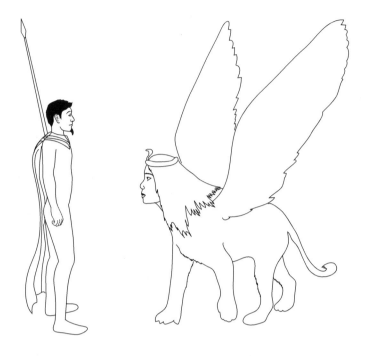

In the famous Greek myth, the hero Oedipus could only continue his journey if he passed the test of the Sphinx who blocked his passage on the road. The test was, of course, a riddle: "What is the animal that has four feet in the morning, two feet at noon, and three in the evening?" Oedipus paused and pondered. Finally he replied, "The animal is man. As a baby he crawls on all fours, as he matures he walks upright on two feet, and in old age he supports himself with a cane." Acknowledging the correct response, the Sphinx granted Oedipus passage.

The picture of perfect alignment I carry in my mind comes from a trip I took to Egypt. I visited the Cairo Museum, Valley of the Kings, rode camels at the pyramids, and saw the Sphinx. But the most vivid impression I remember were the women in the countryside in the more impoverished parts of Cairo. They stood perfectly and looked like the aristocratic figures of the ancient Egyptian kings and queens.

It was even more striking when the women carried baskets on their heads. As I watched, I noticed that even in old age, the load-balancing women retained their erect and regal carriage.

These women seemed to be completely unaffected by the painfully bent posture we associate with elderly people in the West. What interested me even more was the contrast between the Egyptian women and the men. It appeared that the men were shorter, less upright, and much older. They had become the picture of the Sphinx's final chapter of life, bent over and leaning on sticks. I have noticed that in cultures where men and women carry objects on their heads, the contrast is like day and night. Both genders grow tall and upright, maintaining excellent posture as the aging process unfolds.

When I left Egypt that time, I took a bus from Cairo through the Sinai desert and into Israel. During the trip from Cairo to the border of Israel, I thought a lot about the Egyptian women balancing objects on their heads. Later, as I slept, I had a crazy dream in which the Sphinx appeared. She asked me a riddle, "What is the answer to staying upright as old age sets in?" I thought about the pictures of past Egyptian queens and pharaohs wearing high headdresses, perfectly balanced. I answered loudly: "Do not get ahead!"

After I woke, it took me a while to get my bearings, but when I did, my thoughts and feelings returned to my dream and the answer to the Sphinx's riddle. I realized that the head sits on top of the body and, just as when it's balancing a book or a basket on top, the head needs to stay in balance over the shoulders and pelvis. When the head is in front of the body, the muscles in the neck and upper body contract to keep your head in that position. As such, "getting ahead" means setting yourself off balance.

Once we arrived at our destination in Tel Aviv, I started to experiment. I placed a book and other objects on my head and walked around my hotel room. After balancing the book while standing, walking, and sitting, I was pleasantly surprised by how right this new balancing practice felt in my body.

## Whatever You Do, Don't Get Ahead

We have certainly heard the directive, "Get ahead!" many times. However, when it comes to posture, what I propose is the polar opposite: Whatever you do, don't get ahead! Often, our posture is such that our heads are trying to get somewhere before the rest of us. This head-leading tendency creates a lifelong habit of leaning forward. When your head leans forward, you take the weight away from the stronger muscles along your spine and legs and redistribute it into the weaker muscles of your neck and upper back. These weaker muscles strain to keep your head upright. This contracting posture also constricts circulation to the spinal column and the head, causing tension in the back and neck. So do not let your head lead the way—that is what legs are for!

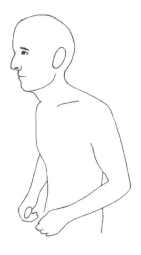

### *The Head-Pelvis Connection*

When we are aligned correctly, the natural position of our bones and joints allows the body's weight to be carried by the strongest muscles. The thighs are many times stronger than the back and are designed to support the lower back by assisting with weight distribution. The thighs tie into the pelvis, which is the connector between the upper and lower halves of the body.

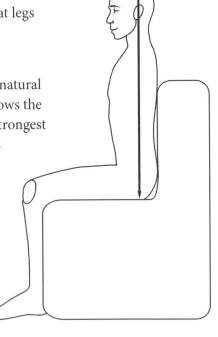

We move by groups of muscles contracting and releasing. When weak muscles take on prolonged weight due to bad alignment, this contracts the muscles and limits range of motion. It also weakens the strong muscles that are designed to take on the main weight of the body. As the saying goes, "If you don't use it, you'll lose it." The strong muscles in the lower back and thighs are not receiving the upper body weight; instead, that weight is distributed into the shoulders, neck, torso, and abdomen. If we maintain this type of alignment, our physical structures slowly cave in on us, which impedes our breathing and our overall health.

Conversely, when you move from your pelvis, the stress of your weight is distributed more evenly throughout your muscles and joints, avoiding undue pressure on any particular region. When your head is lined up over your pelvis, your weight is naturally distributed, supporting a more balanced body frame. This balance extends all the way up to the head and all the way down to the feet. The main principle here involves keeping your head's center of gravity lined up with that of your body, especially the shoulders and pelvis. When we learn to align the head with the pelvis, we fall into a natural posture, and we no longer engage in an unconscious fight with gravity. It is a very easy process, though it may take some conscious awareness and effort at first to re-educate and realign your body. Proper alignment is a pleasurable sensation. Finding it involves hearing and experiencing the body say, "Yes!", as it feels a sense of natural comfort and inner confidence.

To start, try taking a regular check on your posture while going through your daily activities. While you are standing, is your head held high, and is it lined up over your pelvis, knees, and ankles? While sitting, is your head lined up over your shoulders and pelvis? Is your rib cage elevated upward, and is your spine extending to its optimal elevation? Be conscious of how you stand, how you sit, and how you walk and run.

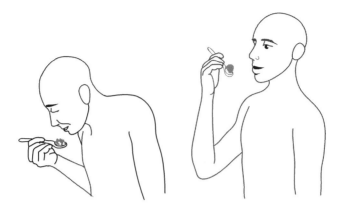

When you're eating, instead of falling into your usual posture, try sitting in extension with your head lined up as much as possible over your pelvis, sit close to the table, and try bringing your food to your mouth instead of the opposite. Be sure to lift your rib cage. Digestion begins in the mouth—chewing well and sitting in an upright position helps move things along more smoothly. Not only that, chewing your food well preps it for your stomach, and it extracts the flavors of your food. Yum!

Developing your consciousness about your posture is the first step toward bringing your body back into balance.

## Seeing Is Believing

The optic nerve has the most direct input into the brain, and for most of us, our sense of reality is formed visually. We don't follow our noses—we actually follow our eyes.

Compared to other species, our sense of smell is a lot less developed than our eyesight. The eye is designed so that, from a standing position, we can look toward the horizon with a natural visual trajectory of 15 degrees downward—this allows us to see what is immediately in front of us. When we bend our heads beyond that 15 degrees, our eyes rotate down and the head and neck bend forward, which eventually leads to strain in our eyes, neck, and other body parts. With the advent of computers, this downward motion and vision has accelerated. The results are clear—for many people, eye, neck, shoulder, and back tension have become the norm.

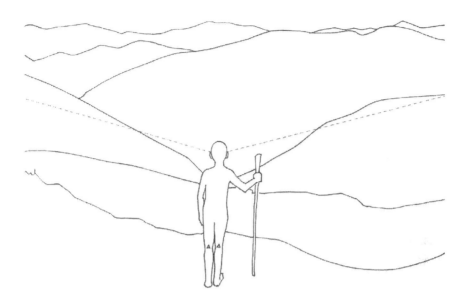

### *Dynamic Alignment Is Easy on the Eyes!*

Changing your posture is good for your entire body, but it's especially good for your eyes. The same way they did back when we were hunters and gatherers, our activities create our posture. These days, people spend a lot of time looking down at close-up objects or screens, and this can cause a great deal of eye strain. It's important, then, to alter your close-up activities with activities that give your eyes a break.

If you find that you are doing one thing too often, like looking down, get up and do the opposite. If your body is in one position, stretch in the opposite direction. For shorter breaks, I like to walk away from my work, go outside, and look at something far away. As you do this, take in the color, shape, and size of that far-away object. Then go back to your close-up visual activity and enjoy better clarity.

When you can take a longer break, one of the best things you can do for yourself is to take a walk and look toward the horizon. When we look toward the horizon, our chins tuck in, promoting a healthier neck curvature. Our shoulders drop and our rib cages gently lift up. It's as if we are back in those days, looking across the horizon for sustenance and observing from afar, just like our ancestors did not so long ago.

In addition to the simple act of taking a walk, the following exercises facilitate good posture and are a pleasant workout for your eyes.

### EXERCISE: *From Tunnel Vision to Peripheral Vision*

Moving and stretching your muscles in opposing ways increases your normal range of motion. This is even true of your eye muscles. This exercise is especially useful for those of us who spend several hours a day looking at a screen.

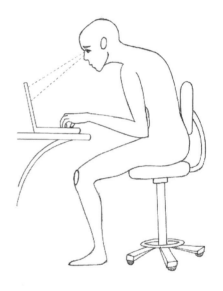

This exercise may seem deceptively simple, but your eyes will thank you for it. It simply requires that you stand up and give your eyes a good stretch. I recommend that you practice this exercise with increasing frequency.

Here's how you do it: Any time you have been narrowly focusing for a while by using a computer, reading, or performing any close-up detail work, go outside, if possible, and allow your eyes to take in the entire horizon. Look as far away as possible.

You can take this exercise further by connecting to your peripheral vision. Soften your eyes and see if you can become aware of what appears on the far edges at the side of you, below you, and above you. After a while, breathe into your eyes. Gently place your hands over your eyes and exhale healing breath energy through the palms of your hands and through your eyes so it fills up your entire being.

Remember that it is within our genetic template to grow upright and look to the horizon. The body was not designed to slump over a laptop, and the eye was not designed to look into a smartphone. So take a break, go outside, and stretch those eyes. Gently bring your shoulders back and extend upward to see what is out there.

**EXERCISE:** *Vision, Breath, Expansion*

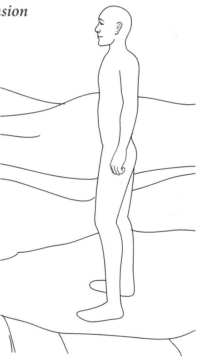

This practice takes the previous exercise a step further. Go to a place where you can clearly see the horizon. Look at a far-away object in the distance and hone in on it. As you inhale, expand your vision outward from that single point to include what you see in your periphery. As you exhale, bring your vision back to that distant focal point. Repeat this vision practice for at least five breaths (but no more than 10) whenever possible. This is a wonderful mood enhancer and is also a refreshing eye exercise for computer users as well as television viewers.

*Standing high, looking afar,
just like our ancestors did*

## Forward Flexion vs. Backward Extension

In chapter three, we began to discuss our human tendency toward flexion, as well as its opposite and countervailing stretch: extension. I cannot emphasize the importance of overcoming flexion enough.

Always remember: A naturally aligned body has better circulation and a heightened capacity to regenerate. One who is properly aligned is less likely to suffer the degenerative breakdown associated with the aging process. Joint degeneration develops in your body over time, and incorrect alignment is quite often the culprit. Over a period of 20 or 30 years of struggling against gravity, conditions such as arthritis, osteoporosis, and muscle and joint diseases are likely to appear. But by modifying our centers of gravity with proper alignment and extension, we preserve our energy and prevent degenerative diseases.

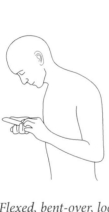

*Flexed, bent-over, looking into a tiny screen*

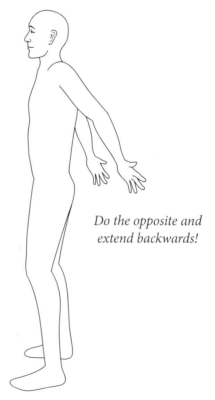

*Do the opposite and extend backwards!*

### *Gravity Got You Down?*

Gravity will make us strong when we are aligned—and it will make us weak when we are not. So, we listen to our bodies, adjust, and chaaa!

Without gravity, we would quickly atrophy. The force of gravity itself is neither positive nor negative—instead, it amplifies our physical patterns. It accentuates our crookedness, and causes problems in the joints and muscles when we are out of alignment. By strengthening our alignment, we can keep ourselves from relying on walkers or canes as we age. Understanding how to tap into the zone of proper alignment can prevent or eliminate the chronic backaches, neck problems, headaches, and other pains that block our energy and make us age more quickly than we should.

When we are upright, gravity tries to pull us down. Test this theory by standing and holding your arms stretched out from your sides. Keep them there. Before long, your arms will become very heavy and, eventually, they will drop. The farther away the parts of your body get from your center, the more difficult it is to resist gravity.

Think of the effects of gravity as a constant workout for your body. A balanced stick will stay upright until a stronger force affects it, but a stick that is not balanced will fall. The human skeleton consists of five groups of bones which are responsible for getting us around and keeping us upright. Like the stick, we must keep these bones in balance.

When these sets of bones work together and stay more extended, or when these bones bend backward and upright, gravity then becomes a strong and helpful friend.

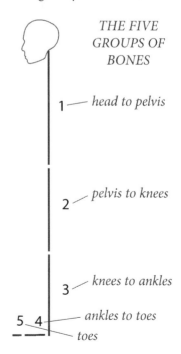

THE FIVE
GROUPS OF
BONES

1 — head to pelvis

2 — pelvis to knees

3 — knees to ankles

4 — ankles to toes

5 — toes

In contrast, when our bones are bending forward, they work against the body's natural balance, and gravity works against us. When we are bending forward, the muscles contract more, and then stay that way in order to stop us from falling forward.

Balanced posture is the result of the body's balanced relationship with gravity. By learning to balance properly, you prevent unnecessary strain on your body. When you practice extension, your head naturally lifts upward and finds its proper position over your neck, shoulders, and pelvis. The spine leans back, bringing your chest upward, stretching the frontal muscles of the spine, and relaxing the muscles along the back of the spine to create more symmetry within the spinal column. This allows for better circulation, improved organ function, and greater physical comfort and ease. Most importantly of all, extension lifts the rib cage and opens up the heart—a physical action that helps us reach the fullest and healthiest life experience.

In terms of the optimal structure and function of the body, you must understand and implement these simple but important principles of flexion versus extension. Consider that the average person spends over 90 percent of his or her time in a bending position. We sit and stand in a forward position for most of every day, and if we are not lying on our stomachs while sleeping, we are most likely sleeping in a bent position as well. As such, work on consciously leaning backward in extension rather than allowing yourself to automatically lean forward. If the concept of leaning backward carries a negative connotation for you, look at it in terms of extending toward the sky, growing tall, opening up and expanding rather than closing in on yourself and struggling against gravity and the world. Good posture denotes energetic self-confidence, a physical balance of strength, and an aesthetic sense of grace and beauty that we can feel on the inside and see on the outside.

Proper physical balance will literally carry you through life, helping you grow toward strong alignment and regeneration.

## Posture: Another Mood Enhancer

A balanced posture is also great for your mental and emotional health. Many of my patients have told me that when they made physical adjustments, their mental and emotional states improved. Why is this so? It happens because the brain is a big sponge that needs a lot of circulation. When the physical body is aligned, it is more open, allowing circulation to move more freely, especially to the brain. In a nutshell, opening up your physical body with a balanced posture allows for healthier brain function, which results in higher levels of the "happy chemicals" I mentioned earlier. As such, good posture definitely enhances a good mood.

When we incorporate the principles of a balanced flexion and extension into our daily activities, we do not slouch as much. When we hold to the principle of extension, we stay balanced because we keep the weight of our bodies more evenly directed toward the strong muscles of the buttocks and thighs. The weight no longer stays so much in the neck and upper back, which receives the weight of our head when the head leans forward. While upright, remind yourself to keep your head over your pelvis as much as possible. By doing so, you are reversing the constrictive forward-bending tendency so you can see from a higher-up perspective. You are lifting your rib cage to open your lungs and heart so you can breathe more freely, and you are allowing yourself to see more and feel better, both mentally and physically.

## EXERCISE: *Flexion and Extension, Forward and Back*

The simple and powerful theme of this exercise is to do the opposite of what we normally do. Extension practices are very simple and effective ways to counteract the adverse effects of habitual flexion, and direct the spinal column toward a more upright posture. These methods are designed to strengthen and lengthen the muscles along the spine and frontal torso, lift the rib cage, and bring the head and pelvis back into alignment. When performed regularly, they counteract our forward-leaning habits and eventually help correct them.

*Muscles in the front and back side of the spinal column*

By lifting the rib cage, we become more upright and take the pressure off our internal organs, facilitating digestion and respiration.

Stand with your knees slightly bent and hips positioned comfortably over your ankles. Place your hands on the top portion of your buttocks with your fingers pointing down. Bring your shoulder blades back and imagine them pointing downward toward your ankles. Drop your chin so as not to put any unnecessary strain on your neck.

Stay in this posture for a while. Remember to breathe and feel comfortable in this new posture. You will notice that it brings your chest out, creating a stronger, more confident presentation to the world.

### Creative Extension

There are so many creative ways to go into extension. Because we all have different body types and needs, explore your own way of extending upward, feeling the stretch along the frontal spine, observing the sensation of lifting your rib cage and enjoying the full depth of your breath. Ever notice the natural comfort of your neck's curvature expanding as you take in a fuller vision? A simple adjustment can make the eventual difference between a healthy, upright body and one that requires a walker.

*Hands on buttocks, chin tucked in, slightly-bent knees, shoulders back and breathe*

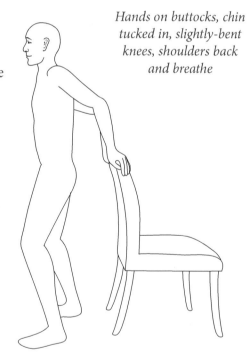

*Instead of sitting in the chair, be creative. Do the opposite and extend.*

Additionally, you can weave the practice of extension into your everyday activities. Simply stand or sit in a balanced posture and extend your spine until you find yourself in a slight, comfortable backbend.

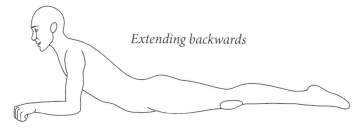

*Extending backwards*

Here's one way you can take time in for a creative extension: Lie on your stomach on the floor. Take a breath and, as you exhale, gently prop yourself up on your elbows. For two to four minutes, focus on your relaxed, rhythmic breath, and let go. If there is any tension in your lower back, try just resting your head on your arms while focusing your breath into the area of tension, and, each time you exhale, focus on letting the tension go.

Remember to adjust into extension when you are eating, sitting, reading, and walking. You may want to imagine the tips of your ears being lifted up. A more common focus is to feel as if something or someone is gently lifting you from your crown while you keep your chin tucked inward and your eyes ahead.

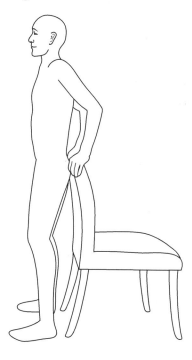

*Standing close to the chair, use the chair to extend your shoulders back, lift your ribcage and slowly breathe.*

Extension increases your lung capacity, relieves physical tension, allows your body to function as it was designed to, and will even make you feel taller. However you extend, the sky is the limit.

## EXERCISE: *Fuller Extensions*

In this next exercise, stand with your back against the side of your bed. Position yourself so that you can gently lean back over the bed. Be sure to use your hands to grip the bed as you crouch down.

Gently lean back with your legs bent accordingly, until you are in a comfortable backbend. Your body should be in the form of an upside-down L shape. As you lean back, cradle the base of your skull with one hand, or use both. If you have a free hand, use it to support yourself as necessary. Breathe and just chaaa for one to three minutes. When you're ready to release this posture, gently and slowly slide down the side of the bed toward the ground.

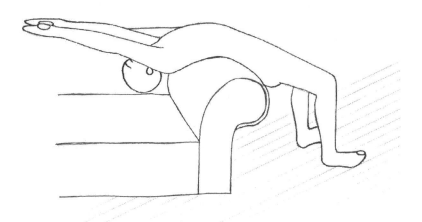

*Leaning over a couch or a bed, stretching backwards
into extension. Don't forget to breathe!*

A final word on flexion and extension: We spend at least 90 percent of our lives in flexion, so be sure you're counteracting the effects of flexion by finding time in your active day to stretch backward and extend your head upward to the sky.

## EXERCISE: *The Book Walk*

For this exercise, balance a book on your head for a moment, and then bring your head forward. Be ready to catch the book because, once your balance is gone, the book slides off.

Balancing a book on your head is a method you can practice to bring your head back into its natural alignment with your spine, facilitating a more healthy body weight distribution, and counteracting the effects of gravity on your posture. You will need a chair or bench of some kind. As you are doing the exercise, notice how your body positions itself as you maintain alignment, distributing your weight onto the strong muscles of your thighs and buttocks.

Begin in a standing position with your chair nearby, and balance a book on the crown of your head. While maintaining your balance with the book still centered on the crown of your head, notice how your chin naturally tucks in to support the natural curvature of your neck. Keeping your shoulders relaxed, slowly sit into your chair.

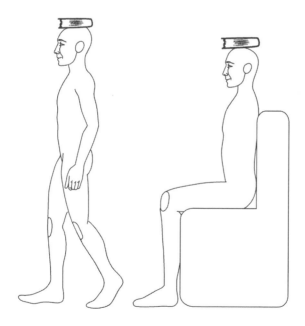

*Imagine your head being a book. Keeping the bookhead balanced over your body while sitting, standing and moving from point A to point B, will naturally align the head-pelvic connection.*

Notice that when the book stays on your head, your upper body and head are more upright and aligned over your pelvis. Your upper body weight is distributed into your body's central physical strength, namely the upper thighs and pelvis. Take a few natural breaths. Stand, walk, and sit feeling aligned and centered. While on the computer, try balancing a book or something else on your head, just like I am now!

## EXERCISE: *Don't Let the Water Spill*

The pelvic core is a group of muscles consisting of four muscle groups shaped somewhat like a basin. The base muscles in this area, called the pelvic floor, are a network of muscles that connect to the front of the body at the pubic bone and fan across, attaching to the pelvis and tailbone on the back side. The pelvic floor is like a net at the base of your trunk that holds your organs and secures your pelvis and lower back. The multifidus muscle secures our backsides from the lower back, hugging the spinal column all the way up to the upper neck; and it works with the pelvic floor and the abdominal muscle to keep the lower back and pelvis stable. The transversus abdominis muscle is the deepest of the abdominal muscles; it spreads across the abdomen, functioning like a corset that holds the pelvis and lower back together. The thoracic diagraphm muscle fans across the top of the three muscles, which holds the top part of the pelvic core acting somewhat like a lid. All four of these muscles act in unison to help secure your structural base, and keep your torso erect.

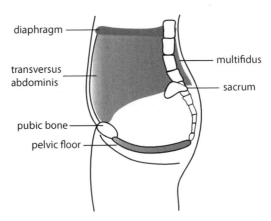

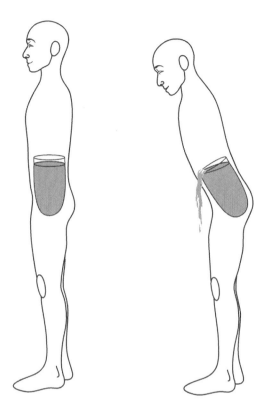

*An erect torso keeps the water from spilling out.*

*When the torso bends, the water spills.*

Imagine the pelvic core as a basin of water. When the basin is level, the water is still. When you slouch forward, or lean onto one leg and let your hips tilt sideways, the water spills. Your objective is not to spill the water. When we figuratively, "spill water," our bodies redistribute the weight of our torsos to its weaker muscles, primarily to the upper body muscles. Simply imagining a level basin of water in your lower torso keeps your back, torso, and head upright, bringing your bones and muscles into a more comfortable alignment. This practice is especially helpful while standing and sitting but not, of course, while lying down.

## EXERCISE: *Roll Walking*

> *"The sovereign invigorator of the body is exercise,*
> *and of all the exercises walking is the best."*
>
> – Thomas Jefferson

Humans are one of only a few species that travel on two legs. And most of us walk thousands of steps every day. Proper walking will alleviate back pain, and even correct chronic conditions, such as lower back and joint stiffness, improving your circulation in the process. Since many of us walk with our minds already where we are heading, our heads are perched out in front of us, as if we are mentally running to where we are going. Remember, the better approach is to move from your lower body. Consciously keeping your head aligned causes gravity to automatically keep your body upright and channels your weight into the stronger muscles of your thighs and buttocks.

Many people stomp and clomp when they walk, but walking should be more of a rolling step than a clonking step. When you walk, roll into your ankles, all the way across the balls of your feet to the tips of your toes. Then begin the process again. This naturally facilitates a fluid weight distribution into the ankles and the joints of the foot, along with the rest of your body. As you walk, remind yourself to walk with a light gait, staying conscious of the terrain you are on.

Remember to step from heel to toe in a calm, gentle manner while you roll your weight from your ankle to the ball of your foot, feeling the roll as you gently make your way from here to there.

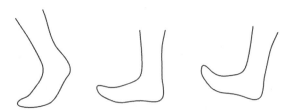

*While walking, roll onto the heel, then onto the ball,*
*then the tips of the toes while taking off into the next step.*
*It is more of a rolling action than a stepping action.*

**EXERCISE:** *Baby Stretch*

A baby stretch is the most natural type of stretch. When babies spontaneously stretch, they involve their whole bodies. There is so much we can learn about breathing and posture from babies. By practicing baby stretches regularly, we, as adults, can tap into that child energy for greater integration of flexibility and respiration. This exercise is great before meditation, after, or even during.

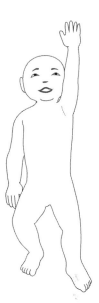

Babies know
how to stretch

In a reclining position, stretch your arms up over your head and reach in both directions from the center of your body. As you inhale, stretch your extremities from your shoulders to your finger tips and from your hips to your toes. When you reach the end of your exhale, pause briefly and hold your stretch. As you exhale, stretch even further, and then release. Release further and chaaa.

## Your Body Already Knows

Babies start off with their own genetic blueprints of knowing what to eat, how to fully breathe, and how to live with excellent posture. Most adults, however, have postural issues. Life is built upon a progression of acquired habits. Children copy what they see, especially in their parents. If the adults have been slouching in a couch, sitting incorrectly for a lifetime, the children will copy these habits and model themselves after what they see. So, if we break our own patterns of bad posture, maybe our children will be less likely to adopt them!

### *Bad Posture by Design*

Prolonged improper sitting is by far the worst thing you can do for your back. Most of us spend a great deal of time sitting. We often sit at work, and even if we do not have a sitting job, we drive home sitting, only to arrive and slouch down on the couch. People who sit for long periods of time invariably develop bad posture, and many are unaware of the head-pelvis connection. Due to this type of chronic sitting, your body starts to lean forward. And, as we discussed earlier, this orientation will eventually distort the integrity of the discs, ligaments, and muscles of your spine.

If you suffer from back discomfort or pain, part of it may be attributed to the designs of your chairs or sofa. Faulty seat design is found everywhere—in homes, the work place, and the vehicles we ride in. The aesthetic design of cheap chairs is often so appealing, that we neither notice, nor think about the effects they could have on our bodies.

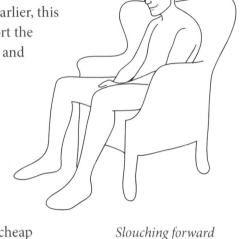

*Slouching forward*

Chairs and couches rarely provide support for the neck and lower back. The best thing while working is to stand and move around as much as possible. If standing is not an option at the workplace or in your home, and you have a chair that contributes to bad posture, you may want to get rid of it. If that is not an option, you will need to improvise. A rolled-up towel or pillow comfortably positioned behind your mid-back will provide more extension. If you have lower back issues, you may want to experiment by positioning the towel at the base of your spine. When you sit, remember to keep your head over your pelvis as much as possible. If you divert from this head-pelvis balance, simply bring yourself back into it as soon as you become aware of it.

When you are sitting, your knees should be level or slightly below your hips. When the seat of a chair is too high, your knees are pushed below the hips, creating a pronounced spine curvature known as a "swayback." When the knees are higher than the hips, the lower back is flattened, thus forming a straight back posture. Both of these sitting issues can lead to constricted muscles, cramped joints, and blocked circulation.

When sitting for long periods, remember the principle of opposites for balance—periodically get up and do the opposite of sitting. Because sitting is a stationary, flexed position, the body is bent forward. To counteract this, stand up and practice the Flexion and Extension, Forward and Back exercise. Bend your knees slightly and place both hands on your buttocks, then bring your body backward into an extension. It is always beneficial to include a good body shake afterward, just to shake out the adverse effects of prolong sitting. You can do this any time, while lying down or even sitting. Simply take a deep inhale and shake on your exhalation.

## Stretching after Vigorous Exercise

As an enthusiastic soccer player, I have found that sitting on the couch after a game invariably stiffens up my back. While many people believe that exercise causes stiffening, that tension or stiffness is usually the result of not stretching, and choosing to sit in a poor or unsupported seated position after vigorous activity.

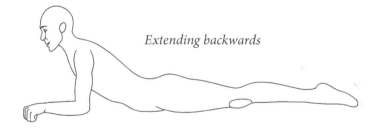

*Extending backwards*

Why is this so? The reason is because exercise loosens the joints. When we sit or slouch in one position for too long, we distort the alignment of the loosened joints, causing inflammation and pain to and around them. When you sit after exercise, your body cools down in a forward position, which contributes to bad posture and to feeling more pain the next day. Instead, the best thing to do after vigorous exercise is to stretch.

After exercise, try extending by lying on your stomach on the floor and use your elbows to slightly prop yourself up, extending your shoulders and head back (the same practice mentioned earlier in the Creative Extension section). This backward bending position allows your body to cool down into an upright spine. Or you may try lying on your back with your knees bent for a few minutes. While lying there, periodically do some gentle stretches.

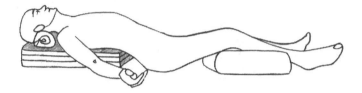

*While lying on your back, prop yourself up so that your chest is elevated and your spine is extended. Don't forget to slowly and fully breathe. Enjoy the chaaa.*

# CHAPTER SEVEN
## *Stretching and Exercise*

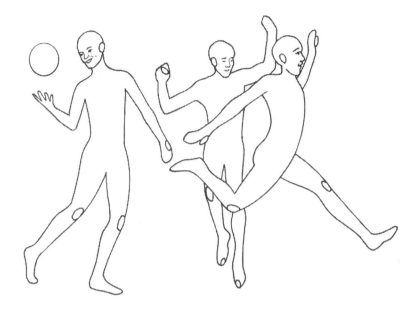

So far, we have spent a great deal of time discussing yin breath, but we can also set aside time for yang breathing and activity in our lives. The best example of yang breath is aerobic breathing. This is when the heart rate increases as the body is in motion. At the peak of this type of breathing is the "runner's high." This euphoric sensation is a product of moving and breathing. It is a truly dynamic state in which blood is moving quickly and the lungs are channeling oxygen into the blood, eliminating toxins from the cells. When the whole body is in motion at the same time, a surge of neurochemical activity brings about a sense of invincibility, youth, and high energy.

This feeling can be addictive and is our body's way of keeping us coming back for more exercise! My personal drugs of choice are dance and soccer. I am simply in awe of how the body can go from a passive mode to a very active mode, and I'm even more in awe if I score a few goals! When I am engaged in aerobic activity, I am reminded of why the human physical upright skeleton took this unique shape. This design allows us to engage on a physical level whether we are running, climbing, swimming, or walking. It seems the only thing we cannot do is fly!

Take running for instance. Human beings are capable of going long distances—this has been part of our evolutionary makeup ever since we left the ocean. Originally, we ran to escape wild animals or to chase them down to eat. Later, running became our way of delivering information between villages. Aerobic activity and breathing originates from that part of our evolution.

In today's society, our yang activities have changed. No longer do we need to chase after our food. We pull it from the refrigerator, order a pizza, or we visit the drive-through. Our cars drive us to and from work and the market. Running has become something we associate with organized sports like soccer, basketball, football, rugby, and field hockey—not a way to get around. As a result of these evolutionary changes, many of us only end up getting vicarious aerobic exercise by watching sports on television.

Despite our modern lifestyle choices, we intuitively know that aerobic exercise is good for us, that it is a gift from our evolutionary heritage. How, then, should we relate to aerobic activity in our world of convenience? I would like to suggest something here as a point of consideration. These days many people work out for all the wrong reasons. As the name implies, it is "work." Many of us work out for vanity, or because the doctor tells us to. These are legitimate, secondary reasons to exercise. But what about the simple pleasure of feeling great inside? My personal philosophy on aerobic exercise is to "play out" rather than work out! When we are having fun, our bodies, minds, and spirits are happier. Fun is like a lubricant to the joints and muscles, and, because of that, it helps us prevent injury. When we play, we perform better, and are less likely to hurt ourselves.

Playful physical activity and full, active breaths go hand in hand. When we are physically active, our muscles, joints, and circulation are in rapid motion. This motion strengthens and detoxifies the body by sweating and breathing those toxins out.

## A Good Stretch

A good stretch feels really great, especially when you have been sitting, standing, or lying down for too long. The subtle feelings and satisfaction are both relaxing and stimulating. Stretching is an individual thing, and you can tailor your stretching practices to your particular size, shape, and temperament—and, of course, to what feels good to you and your body.

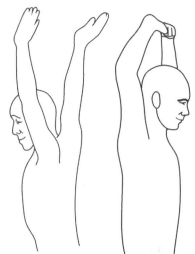

All animals stretch. Have you ever spent the day with a domestic cat? It will stretch slowly several times during the course of the day, thus it maintains its suppleness and flexibility. Similarly, one of the first things we humans do when we wake up in the morning is stretch. This act not only lengthens your muscles, but it also serves to help wake you up! As an adult human, you will notice how great it feels to stretch after you have been in front of a computer, or after you have been sitting or driving for a long time. The reason it feels so good is because the stretch sends blood to the muscles that were still while you sat or drove, and in so doing, the blood brings energy into the muscles— healing energy.

Regular stretching benefits you in many ways. It definitely pays to be more cat-like. Here are some of the benefits you will enjoy by adding more stretching into your daily routine:

- Increased endurance and stamina
- Reduced stress
- Improved flexibility
- Reduction of muscle strain injuries
- Relaxation
- Stimulation of the body's cells, organs, and muscles
- Increased circulation

### How to Stretch

Stretching can be done at any time of day and in any position: while lying down, sitting, or standing, at work, before play, or in a car. Whenever it feels right, do not hold back!

Most people will automatically stretch when they are stiff. However, there is a right way and a wrong way to stretch. The right way is to first consciously feel the area that you are stretching, and to breathe rhythmically as you move slowly and let go. Stretch until you feel a slight pull. Then hold your stretch for five to 10 seconds and release it, all the while maintaining a rhythmic breath. Each time you stretch, try to gently increase your range. Stretch until you feel that resistance or pull, hold, then release, chaaa, and breathe.

The wrong way to stretch is with sudden, fast, or bouncy actions. Also be cautious not to take a stretch too far. Stretching in any of these ways causes the body to react by tightening up, and it can cause injury. Our bodies work much better when we slow down, and stretch in rhythm with our breathing.

### Yoga and Stretch Classes

Yoga and stretch classes have become very common, and there are many different forms of yoga—everything from aquatic to hot yoga. All of these yogic exercises are wonderful if they are performed correctly. If you do not perform them correctly, as with any other type of exercise, they can cause injuries. If you're beginning a new program of yoga or stretch classes, remember to take it slow. Allow yourself some time to be a beginner.

Also keep in mind that the instructor does not know you like you know yourself. Never try to keep up with the teacher—or with others—in your class. If Yogi Joe is next to you performing radical stretch movements, this does not mean you should take it to the same extreme. We all have our own unique strengths and limitations, which is a good thing. So if you attend yoga or stretch classes, strive for sensations that fill your body with a natural sense of "Yes." Rather than overexerting, make the necessary adjustments to achieve a balanced sense of challenge, comfort, and alignment.

## EXERCISE: *Aerobic Breathing, Yang Power*

Here we emphasize the importance of the rhythm of breathing during aerobic activity. Aerobic breathing is deep, rhythmic, and charged with life. Rhythmic breathing provides a smooth distribution of energy which supports a graceful physical expression and endurance.

When you are about to engage in athletic or aerobic activity, begin by taking three deep, relaxed, rhythmic breaths. Allow the breath to be gently pulled in by your muscles, and consciously focus your awareness on that deep breath coming into you. Set your intention to believe in yourself, and have fun. Feel your inner life energy get ready to go active. This is a sure-fire motivator to help you get the best from the coming activity.

On your fourth or fifth breath, start your routine. Warm up and breathe into those body parts you are stretching. It is also great to give yourself a few slaps on the legs, buttocks, and chest to loosen up your muscles and joints. As you do this, notice the rhythmic feeling of your breath. As your breathing muscles move smoothly and your body becomes physically aerobic, stay attuned to that underlying sense of rhythm. Every cell listens to this awareness, as do your heart, lungs, muscles, and your overall being.

Most of us have fun when we play aerobically, and rhythmic breathing definitively enhances the fun! As an over-60 soccer player/enthusiast, I can attest to the value of rhythmic breath while being aerobically active. When I am in rhythm and somebody tackles me, though there may be significant force involved, being in rhythm softens the blow. I am convinced that rhythmic breath not only loosens my muscles, but it also provides more flexibility and resilience to prevent injury. Remember to check in with your rhythm throughout your playtime.

## EXERCISE: *Shake, Rattle, and Roll*

Shaking your body while breathing out
is one of the best ways to release tension
of all kinds: physical, emotional, mental,
and even sexual. It helps to remove
stored-up thought forms and patterns
as well as physical fixations.

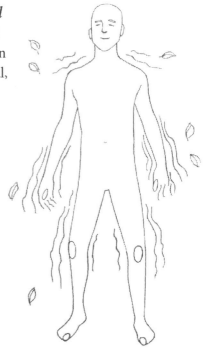

You can practice this exercise
while standing or lying down, but
lying down is best, because it allows
you to really let your body *go*!
Lie down on your back on a bed
or a carpeted floor—somewhere
soft where there is plenty of room.
If you choose to stand, your feet
should be shoulder-width apart,
and your knees should be loose
and slightly bent.

Inhale slowly and deeply. Exhale fully through your nose and release
all the leftover air from your lungs. Remembering to observe the pause,
take another deep breath, and as you exhale, begin to shake your entire
body—like a tree shaking off its dead leaves—until you have exhaled
completely. Breathe in again. "Shake, rattle, and roll" on the exhale.
Go through this exercise until you feel your tension being released.

## EXERCISE: *Shake and Shout*

This exercise is a variation on the Shake, Rattle, and Roll exercise.
Position yourself and start with a full cycle of breath, as you did
before. On your second exhalation, shake, but this time, as you exhale,
make a sound—any sound. Do not worry about the neighbors. Just
let it all out, especially if you are releasing emotional tension. It may
feel ridiculous at first, but after you do this a few times, you will notice
immediate positive results. You can do the Shake, Rattle, and Roll
exercise in tandem with any of the other breathing exercises, or any
time you feel tension creeping up on you.

**EXERCISE:** *The Isolated Shake*

You can apply this therapeutic shaking anywhere: your hands, feet, shoulders, or legs. It feels great to shake your wrists, fingers, and arms after being on the computer for a while, for example. A good leg shake feels great after a long drive. In this variation, pay attention to your individual body parts to create relaxation, and improve your circulation.

Isolate any single body part: a leg, your torso, an arm, etc., and breathe into that body part. On the exhalation, shake and enjoy.

Try shaking from your lower back all the way up to your head and back down again to your feet. Shaking from the sacrum region causes a ripple effect, because the sacrum region is the center of your body. When you feel that ripple, don't be surprised—it simply means you're doing it right!

# CHAPTER EIGHT
## *Touch*

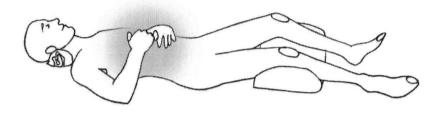

We talked earlier about the ability humans have to heal themselves and others through touch. We intuitively push acupressure points and rub sore muscles. When we are going through both physical and emotional turmoil, we hold ourselves and each other through it. Think of the last time a friend came to you and shared difficult news—one of your first inclinations was, most likely, to reach out and touch or hug your friend.

Throughout the animal kingdom, touch is a common necessity. If a newborn calf is not licked by its mother, that calf will most likely die. A human baby who is not held and nurtured will grow up to feel insecure and unwanted. Human beings need the same things as all other mammals—to be touched, nurtured, and loved. When you have a cramp in your leg or foot, or tightness in your muscles, you automatically press on the area to alleviate the tension and pain. This is certainly nothing new. Human beings have evolved over millions of years, and the innate intelligence within all of us instinctively guides us to press or feel around an injury. When you massage and soothe a stiff muscle, feel around for a possible broken bone, or even just randomly touch a spot that feels good, you begin a process of healing energy transmission. The hands assess the body's needs in order to begin the healing process.

> *"Often the hands will solve a mystery that the*
> *intellect has struggled with in vain."*  – Carl Jung

## Relearning How to Heal

Your body's knowledge of how to heal through touch is clearly linked to instinct. And truly, our cells know better than we think. Bruce Lipton, PhD, author of *The Biology of Belief*, cites a study on muscle cells to demonstrate this. In this study, researchers removed muscle cells and placed them in a Petri dish and then added toxins. By the next morning, the cells had migrated as far away from the toxins as possible. Next, the toxins were removed and replaced with nutrients. The following morning, the colony of cells had migrated to the nutrients and had begun absorbing them to receive nourishment.

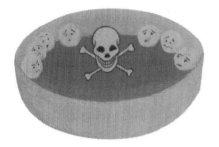 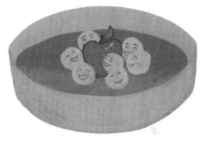

*Cells keeping away from the toxins.*　　　*Cells eating the nutrients. Yum!*

This experiment reflects the intelligence of individual cells—they know what harms and nourishes them. Collectively, all 30 trillion of our cells work as one body that instinctively knows what is best. So as you are relearning how to heal, remember to follow your instincts, and listen to what your body tells you.

## The Healing Touch

One of the most profound early memories I have is of my mother touching me in a way that ignited a feeling of love, energy, and security. She had what I call the healing touch. Without formal training, she knew where to touch and how much pressure to apply. She was very much in tune with her ability to channel energy through her hands to her children. Somehow she knew that this was good for us, and I can testify to that as a recipient of her touch. She was "chaaasome" at it. I have continued her legacy. With my own four children, I realized the importance of good nutrition, freedom of expression, and a healing touch. Touching my children lovingly, whether they were happy, sad, or hurt, has, I believe, been an intricate part of their development.

### *Touch as First Aid*

I have used the combination of touch and breathing as first aid a number of times. One day a couple of years ago, as I was bouncing on the trampoline in my yard with my nephew and two other children, I slipped and fell between the springs. I felt an immediate and severe pain in my ankle. My first reaction was 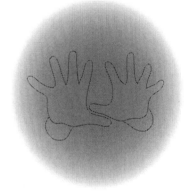 fairly primal: "Oh shit, I don't need this right now." I was scheduled to travel the next day to meet a longtime patient in Europe, and I could not visualize myself working on crutches. I grabbed the throbbing and swelling ankle and began projecting healing breath into it. As I continued to press hard through my hands, I could feel the pain beginning to subside. After I repeated the treatments throughout the day and evening, my ankle stabilized. I was able to make the trip without major disruption, a cane, or crutches.

## *Healing Breath Touch on a Spinal Cord Injury*

On one particular Tuesday evening while soaking in the bath, I received a telephone call from a pastor at UCLA Medical Center. My former wife, Katherine, had been in a very serious accident and was close to death. I immediately rushed to the UCLA Medical Center and arrived just as she was being wheeled out of the emergency room to the MRI. At that time, we did not know the exact extent of her injuries. We did know that she had traumatized her spinal cord. She had lost all mobility and sensitivity from the neck down. As she was wheeled down the hospital corridor, I placed my hands over the site of the injury and projected healing breath touch into the traumatized tissues.

When she returned to the critical care bed, her three children, as well as some close friends, all became involved. Under my instruction, we all took a quick inhalation through our noses and then, breathing out slowly through our mouths, visualized the breath going out, through our hands and into Katherine's body.

Soon after this, she could feel again, although she still had no mobility. When she could finally talk, she said, "I distinctly felt the healing being projected into me. Things became so vivid that the healing projected by David allowed me to feel safe and secure. I also felt very close to death, and the healing energy drew me back toward life. I felt energy going to my injury, creating a deep healing."

Katherine sustained multiple fractures to her spinal cord. She was placed in traction to reset the dislocation in her neck. She then underwent two operations in which her surgeons removed fragments of broken bone, grafted a piece of her hipbone onto her neck, and then screwed it all together with titanium plates.

Before and immediately after the operation, I applied healing breath and touch treatments aimed at reducing the swelling and reestablishing the nerve pathways. One doctor commented that if she had received such an injury only 15 years ago, she would have died. But her operation was a complete success. When the neurosurgeon's work was complete, Katherine's case followed standard protocol, which then included rehabilitation. In almost all cases, healing breath touch is not included in this, however after many conversations with the medical staff, I was able to work with her.

I treated her sometimes two or three times a day. Two and a half years after the event, this is what Katherine has to say: "I have made a remarkable recovery. I am walking, driving, and living an active life. A lot of it had to do with David's unique healing involvement. I wish that this method was available to all of the unfortunate people who injure their spinal cords, because I know what a difference it makes."

### Breathing into Trauma – The Story of Jahcai

In August of 2009, my youngest son, Jahcai, was struck by a car. The accident resulted in a head fracture with internal bleeding. Both the tibia and fibula in his left leg were also broken. When I first arrived to the emergency room, he was semiconscious and quite confused. His head injury caused swelling inside his skull, which produced great pain. The doctors were not sure if he had sustained injury to his spinal cord, so they put a collar on his neck, but even in his semiconscious state, he tried pulling it off!

I spoke to him and told him everything would be OK, and reminded him to breathe into the pain. Later, his mother Heidi arrived and we both stayed with him. Jahcai received several CT scans throughout the night to monitor his bleeding. The doctors were very concerned about brain hemorrhaging. I sat with him all night, projecting my breath, touch, and energy into his head. Around 4 a.m., the CT scan revealed that his internal bleeding had halted.

Later on, he was taken to the critical care unit where he spent the next six days. He was monitored and observed 24 hours a day. The first four days were very rough for Jahcai, and in his semiconscious state, he tried pulling off the electrodes that had been placed on his head to monitor his brain function. When friends and family came to visit, I asked that they not speak to Jahcai, but rather lay their hands on his body, breathe through their noses, and project the exhalation of their breath energies through their hands and into his body.

The nurse assigned to monitor my son said that in all her years of critical care she had never seen this type of treatment having such great effect. Jahcai was recovering quickly. When his head injury had stabilized, his left leg was operated on. The procedure required general anesthesia, resetting the bones, installing a metal rod to hold the bones in place and, after that, stitching his leg back up. The operation was a complete success.

After the operation, Jahcai, his sister, Hyacinth, and I were in his room when a group of doctors came in. The doctor in charge asked Jahcai how he was. My son replied, "Fine." The doctor looked at the amount of medication he had taken—it was none. Jahcai had been given a handheld device to administer pain medication whenever the pain levels became too high for him. When the doctor asked why he had not used any medication, Jahcai paused for a moment, looked at the doctor, and said, "I want my own body chemicals to manage my pain."

I could not believe my ears. I thought, "Jahcai, you dance to your own music!"

The doctor and his team also could not believe what they heard. After an awkward moment of silence, the doctor said, "And how exactly do you do that?"

Jahcai replied, "I realize that it's normal to feel pain after such a big operation, so I accept it, breathe into it, and it seems to feel better."

There was another moment of silence. Then, with an authoritative tone, the head doctor said to him, "If you're in pain, your body will not heal properly. Take your medication." And with that, the team of doctors turned around, off to see the next patient.

At the time I thought, "You guys are going to remember this case."

All three of us remained silent for a while. Jahcai eventually said, "Later on tonight, I'll take some of the medication and it will help me sleep."

My reply was, "Fair enough."

When I reflect on that period, I realize that, instead of using the normal quota of medication, Jahcai opted to use directional breathing—breathing into the pain—and the healing touch given by his friends and family. And it worked.

Healing touch increases the circulation of blood, lymph, nerve stimulation, and microelectric circuits or chi. In this way, healing touch renews the body's circulation to these constricted or traumatized areas, thereby reopening the vital flow of life.

## Breaking Blockages the Yin Way

The hands are a medium that transfer and receive energy. As much as the hands give, the body receives. The body also gives, while the hands receive. Simply being aware of the flow of energy between the hands and the body brings you into a deeper tactile awareness of your overall healing energy. Any time you touch yourself, you are being touched back by your body. This awareness brings us into a full sense of self that allows us to feel a blissful calmness from deep within our cores. This awareness is there to be enjoyed; after all, we are energetic beings. Touching is a medium to experience this healing energetic source.

Pressing is one of the oldest reflexes in our genetic memory. Through inquisitive pressure, we become self-diagnostic. Pressing allows us to search out and probe underlying blockages such as muscle tension, painful joints, tense organs, and underlying emotional feelings, especially in the abdominal area. Believe it or not, pressing and breathing into pain and discomfort can actually produce feelings of pleasure and well-being, allowing us to air out our discomforts and chaaa. Developing tactile sensitivity allows us to find out about the inner workings of our underlying feelings and body parts.

There is a tremendous advantage to learning how to touch yourself in a healing, loving way. You sense better than anyone when you have pressed on a point of tension because you are the one living in your body! You can intuitively feel when your body is sending you signals to press more deeply, or to back off a bit.

The purpose of combining touch and breath, is to transmit directive breath energy through tactile touch into the tissues. The combination of touch and breath re-establishes vital circulation within the body. With that circulation comes healing. This is yet another way we can remove the blockages in our circulatory systems, leaving us free to enjoy good health and vitality. If we don't break the blockages, a dis-ease in the body's vital flow occurs, causing stress to build in the muscles, organs, and entire body, which stresses you even more. It's not only disease or injury that creates these blockages—our negative thoughts can create them, too.

Sadly, it seems universal that we all obsess on thoughts. When you are actively obsessing about something, you probably find that you hold your breath and tense up—this begins the process of creating blockages that interfere with the flow of your circulation. There are many approaches to breaking these blockages—remember that the yang way includes exercise and aerobic activity. We all know that aerobic exercise is healthy, but some blockages require a different kind of healing—the yin way.

This approach includes lying still, entering a chaaa state, and using breath and touch to stimulate your inner circulation away from the tense muscles, and into your organs and internal life energy. When we can take a little time in during the day to yin-ify—or go inward—the rest and rejuvenation allows us to find the energy that comes from a deeper source of awareness. As you practice your healing touch, be light and gentle with yourself when necessary, and go deeper when you need to get more intimate with your muscles and aches.

Accordingly, nature has given special attention to our hands. Enriched with nerves and blood vessels, hands are incredibly sensitive. The hands are powerful receptors, transmitting information and energy.

The powers of touch and breath can channel energy into your underlying tissue, which then becomes warmer. In addition, the electromagnetic changes stimulate the nerves that give feedback to the brain, which in turn elevates neurotransmitter production, resulting in an overall sense of well-being.

You can guide yourself through an exploration of the points that are most relevant to your particular condition by using a two-part process that involves performing a full body scan, and applying pressure with your healing hands. When you perform any of the pressure exercises in this book, the exercises you choose, as well as their duration, is entirely up to you. Do them until you feel a natural sense of satisfaction, or until you feel balance attained in your body. You can then choose to move on to another area, or just go forward with your day!

**EXERCISE:** *Finding and Releasing Stress with Light Pressure*
First, lie on your back in a comfortable position and take a deep, regular breath. Feel the breath going into your body. Focus on only your breath for about five cycles of breath. Next, on an inhalation, follow your breath through your body, making a slow journey from head to foot.

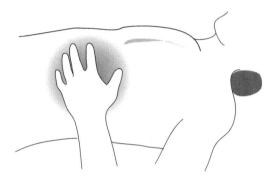

Observe how you feel. Which muscles are tense? When you encounter a tight muscle, contract it once, and then let the tension go, as you breathe through it and let the muscle expand. Take mental note of each part of your body where you feel any tightness, pain, discomfort, or tension, and repeat the process of contracting and breathing into each of those muscles.

Once you have completed this full body scan, let your hands gravitate to one of the places on your body where you recognized discomfort. Apply light pressure over the area, following your instincts. Listen to your body and allow it to guide you. Gradually sink just a little deeper into the pressure and the underlying feelings, while you breathe into the area. When you find tender places, your body is asking you to spend additional time there. As you apply pressure to these areas, be aware of the sensations in your palms and fingers, and feel the tactile connection of the skin your hands are touching, and the deeper underlying energies there. This light laying on of hands creates a synergy between the body, breath, and healing touch, bringing with it a renewal of your body's vital circulation and an overall sense of inner openness.

As you practice, you will become more familiar with yourself. You will begin to recognize areas that hold discomfort, and you will also learn from feeling parts of your body that are very comfortable to the touch. Often, a light touch brings with it a deep experience, and a sense of overall relief.

### EXERCISE: *Finding and Releasing Stress with Deep Pressure*
We are like bodies of water that need to move. The more we move our internal waters, the healthier we become. Here, breathing into deep pressure allows access to blockages in the muscles and deeper levels of circulation. Applying deep pressure as you exhale, your body becomes more open to the accompanying sensations. This exercise is especially good for old injuries or for releasing old emotional baggage.

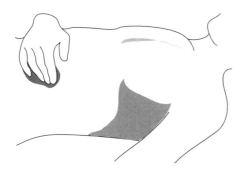

Take a comfortable sitting, lying, or standing position. Start with a relaxed, regular, slow, deep breath. Scan your body for an area of discomfort, a blockage, or pain. Lightly press into this area over four to five cycles of regular, deep breath. Breathe directly and deeply into the painful area. Be sure not to force your breath. Try not to resist the pressure you apply to the area. In your mind's eye, let the pressure melt and dissolve the underlying spasms or blockages in your body.

As you inhale, ease up on the pressure. As you exhale, go deeper. As you breathe in, decrease the pressure again. This pattern of inhaling while easing the pressure and exhaling, while applying deeper pressure, makes use of your body's natural tendency to release tension. Your body already wants to let go—this exercise helps move that desire along.

As you practice this, breathe and press into the belly (the center) of the pain, allowing the pressure to follow your breath. Spend a few cycles of breath there, and then, after a while, back way off. Gently touch the area, feeling your channel of breath energy as it acts as an internal release and a topical analgesic.

Learn to trust yourself, and the wise messages your body gives you, as you practice this exercise. If your body says you're applying too much pressure, listen and ease up. If your body says "Yes!" when you apply deep pressure, try gently increasing it.

### EXERCISE: *Healing Breathing Hands*

There is a synergy between breath and touch; two things that we are naturally doing all the time. Applying touch to a painful or tense area while exhaling is an amazing way to channel breath energy through our hands and into the underlying body parts. Using the breath-press method will arouse your sensory perception, and send powerful healing signals throughout your body that will enhance your overall state of well-being.

When you practice the breath-press method, you draw healing energy in through your nose, and slowly exhale it through your mouth, while visualizing that healing energy moving out through your hands, as you press into an area of your body.

Begin by sitting, lying, or standing comfortably. Place your hands on any part of your body. Be aware of the sensations in your palms and fingers, and then notice the sensation of the skin your hands are touching. Now take a deep inhale through your nose, and slowly exhale through your mouth. In your mind's eye, visualize the breath going out through your hands. Be sure not to grab your breath from your upper body, but instead, breathe from your lower breathing muscles and allow your breath to flow in deeply and smoothly.

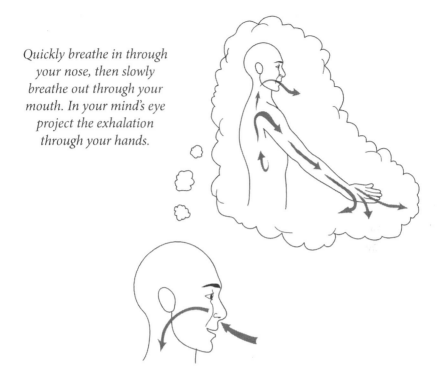

*Quickly breathe in through your nose, then slowly breathe out through your mouth. In your mind's eye project the exhalation through your hands.*

Repeat several cycles of breath this way, visualizing your exhales as healing energy you are directing back into your body through your hands. As you do this, you are extracting the atmosphere and channeling it through your hands into whatever area you are touching. Your body is responding to the placement of your hands by changing the electromagnetic frequency in that area. This change stimulates your circulatory, nervous, and lymphatic systems. The vessels dilate and circulation increases, producing a pulse. This pulse is actually not pumped directly from the heart. It is a local pulse created by its own vascular neuroelectrical system. Breathing and touching stimulate the local circulation, and that creates a ripple effect that benefits the entire body. It is a chaaa connection.

**EXERCISE:** *Touch as a Depression Antidote*

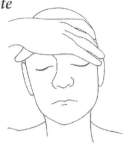

For many of us, it's our automatic response to press on our foreheads when we feel depressed or anxious, and this is an excellent impulse. These points stimulate our ability to think clearly. This powerful practice helps you immediately reduce depression in a very short time.

Lie down on your back and lay your forearm across your forehead just above the bridge of your nose. In this position, your arm contacts most of the acupressure points across the forehead that are often used to treat depression. One of these points is called the third eye point, which is located on the midline slightly above the inner end of the eyebrows. This gland converts photons (sun energy) into body energy, and influences the brain and the hypothalamus, which is sometimes called the master gland.

As you lie there with your forearm across your forehead, feel the weight of your hand and arm as it rests there, gently covering your closed eyes. This calming effect stimulates and releases pressure points relating to your brain's frontal lobe.

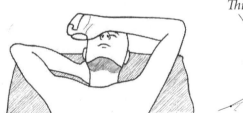
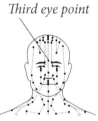
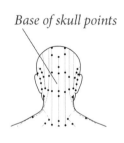

*Third eye point*   *Base of skull points*

Meanwhile, place your other hand along your upper neck at the base of your skull. As you feel the pressure, concentrate on the natural weight bearing down on your third eye, as well as on the other points across your forehead. Be aware of the tactile sensation you are experiencing. You may see different colors, and even some light. Focus on the light, as you breathe into the pressure. Concentrate on directing a relaxed, slow, deep, rhythmic breath moving upward into your head. You can practice this method for five minutes or as long as you want.

As you continue to feel the breath ascend from your base into your head, notice how the activation of these points helps you move the circulation in your entire head, allowing depression or anxiety (or both!) to drift slowly away. Try a gentle smile—even a small smile adds to the experience. This practice enhances your mood and produces a happier outlook from within.

## Treating the Opposite Side

Practitioners of Chinese medicine recognize that Carl Jung's principle of opposites applies to everything in nature, including, of course, yin and yang. For every yin acupuncture and acupressure point, there is a yang acupuncture and acupressure point. For every muscle that contracts, a muscle releases. Your body's design is one of balance, and because of that, your healing practices should be balanced, too. So, when you practice healing touch on one side of your body, be sure to treat the same area on the other side of your body as well.

When you apply healing touch to yourself, the newly infused energy in your body can then enter into specific underlying tissues and related organs. Ailing or stagnant organs thus receive the stimulation and support they need to revitalize their functionality.

To take the idea even further, think again about the body's 14 meridians, discussed earlier. Along the body's primary meridians, there are many other meridians that house thousands of acupressure points; these pathways spread in all directions throughout the body.

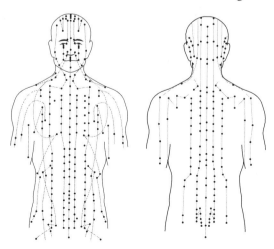

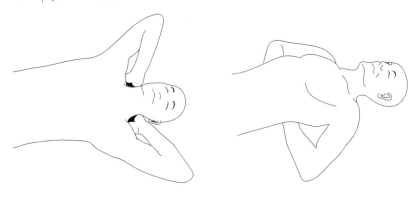

*Lying down on your fists or hand, position your body weight
so that it's pressing into the muscle tension along both sides of the
spine including the neck. Be creative and enjoy the connection!*

Given that, when you touch yourself virtually anywhere on your
body, you are touching pressure points that are connected to your
entire energetic circulatory system. You can help maintain that
interconnected balance in your body by treating both sides any time
you perform healing practices on yourself.

## The Three Burning Spaces

In traditional Chinese medicine, the torso
represents the three burning spaces. The
upper torso represents fire, which includes air,
blood, and the immune system. The middle
torso represents earth, which regulates your
digestion; it is also your emotional center. The
lower torso represents water. This element
regulates your reproductive, urogenital, and
sexual energy. The lower torso includes your
physical center, where your legs attach to your
torso. This is the midpoint between your head
and your feet.

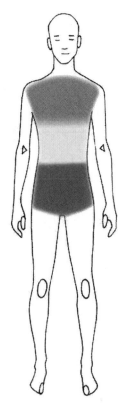

Because these three energy centers
represent such important areas within your
body, it makes sense to learn how to use touch
to heal them.

## Fire

Even when your thoughts are screaming your failings, your heart keeps beating, and the pulse of life continues. You can thank your upper body—and the elements of air and fire—for that. Air is the most immediate life force—the lungs receive it, and the heart delivers it. If you want to fire up your energy and refocus your screaming thoughts, let your healing make contact with the organs of fire.

The upper torso receives air from the atmosphere. It then goes to the heart, which pumps it to every cell in the body. The upper torso also houses the big lymph vessels and thymus gland. Both the lymph and thymus play a vital role in the immune system. Physically, the neck and head sit on the upper torso. When we stretch backward into extension, we open up the fire element. If we couple this with breathing and touch, everything in the upper torso functions a lot better.

## EXERCISE: *Immune Enhancer*

The beneficiaries of the upper torso are the lungs, heart, large lymph vessels, and the thymus gland. The lymph is the front line of defense for the immune system. The big lymph vessels in the upper torso readily respond to gentle touch and pressure, breathing, and chaaa time. The job of the thymus gland (sometimes called the "university" of the immune system) is to produce approximately 10 percent of the elite antibodies designed to eliminate sophisticated viruses and bacteria in the body. The thymus gland, located right under the breast bone, grows until puberty. It then begins the process of shrinking until it no longer has the capacity to produce those antibodies, ultimately compromising the immune system and life force.

An excellent way to loosen the chest region and to stimulate underlying circulation to the inner recipients is to hit on your chest with an open palm, or a closed fist. It is also a great practice for smokers or former smokers, or even city dwellers who breathe in whatever the city's air has to offer their lungs. The shower is a great place to give yourself a few good chest hits.

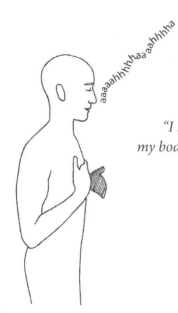

*aaaaaahhhhhaaaahhhha*

*"I like to give this very ancient part of
my body a few good whacks and make sounds:
'aAaaaaaaaahhhhhhahahaha.'"*
– Ringo Starr,
from Dr. Kearney's video,
"Power Healing"

If you wish, do what my friend Ringo Starr likes to do, and make a sound as you exhale. The ancient Jewish doctors recommended hitting oneself on the chest to promote longevity. Five to 10 good slaps stimulate circulation, and can even improve respiration and cardiac function.

This method of beating on the chest is also used by our closest cousins, the monkeys and apes—perhaps they understand something we do not.

### The Heart

As far as amazing organs go, the heart is at the apex. It is a self-regulatory pump that changes its own pace, speeding up or decelerating depending upon your body's overall needs. It is about the size of your fist, yet it is able to pump blood thousands of miles, working day and night throughout your lifetime. This powerhouse is a generator of the largest electromagnetic field in the body, transmitting not only internally, but also externally. Wildly, this force can be measured several feet away from you with a device called a superconductor. The heart's magnetic field is thousands of times stronger than that of the brain!

When your brain and heart are in harmony, it works miracles for your health and well-being. An engaged heart equals lower blood pressure, improved brain function, enhanced neurology, and a calm, quiet demeanor. In a manner of speaking, the mind is the intellect and the heart is the intelligence. When we listen to both the mind and heart, we are wise, in the truest sense.

In traditional Chinese medicine, the organs are described as officials in an empire with the heart as king. It may seem strange to personify the organs in your body this way, but have you heard the tale of a Russian heart donor and the American heart recipient? After the American patient recovered, he could sing Russian songs. So maybe personifying our organs isn't so strange after all!

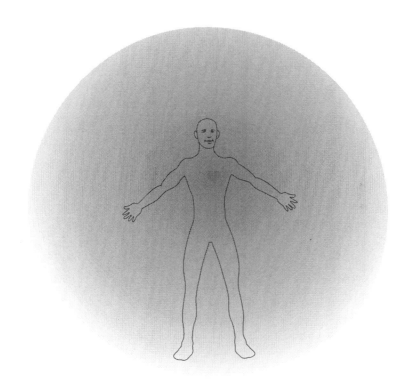

**EXERCISE:** *A Heartfelt Touch*
Your heart will love you when
you send it energy by chaaaing,
pressing, and breathing into
the points that enhance its
function. This next practice
enriches the heart, and
supports the immune and
respiratory systems.

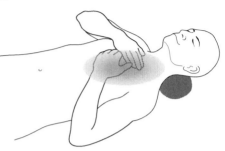

Stand, sit, or lie down. Gently place your right hand over the
upper part of your chest, just below your throat. Position your left
hand over the middle of your chest in line with your nipples. Keep
your hands there for a few moments, breathing through your hands
into your chest. After a while, you will become aware of the warmth
and the tingling sensation being exchanged between your hands and
your body. As you breathe and tune into this energetic and tactile
exchange, your underlying tissues (including your heart, thymus,
lymphatic vessels, and lungs) all gladly receive this energetic tactile
nourishment. Continue this practice as long as you wish. Remember
to focus on a relaxed, rhythmic breath throughout your practice and
enjoy. It really can be quite blissful.

### Earth

In many belief systems around the world, the abdominal region
is considered the source of energetic and physiological power. In
the Chinese system, this part of the torso corresponds to the earth
element, which is interlinked with food, digestion, and energy. In
Japan, the abdomen, called the *hara*, is considered the root of life.
The Japanese believe that by stimulating the hara, we enhance our
precious life force. Some Japanese medical specialists treat only the
abdomen to produce stronger conditions of life and health.

These organs are part of your "factory of life"—they are all main players in the immune and digestive systems, as well as in a myriad of other crucial bodily functions. As such, it is a great idea to give them energy by consciously pressing, breathing, and relaxing into them— particularly in the points under the rib cage. It is common to be sensitive or tender to the touch in this area. When you suffer from digestive problems, these pressure points are usually tense. Therefore, another great way to facilitate digestion is to rub or press your belly after you eat. You see people do this all the time. The human body is instinctively open to a healing touch and cries out, "Yes!", when

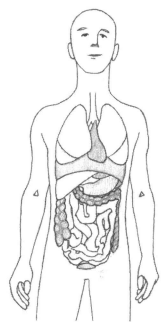

our hands follow the instinct. Next time you finish a meal, try relaxing into slow, natural breathing while you gently rub your tummy. Yum!

## EXERCISE: *Wringing Out Your Emotional Sponge*

The solar plexus is located just below the middle of your rib cage directly up from your belly button. It is like a sponge that absorbs feelings. Most of us know the phrase, "I felt it in my gut." In actuality, you felt it in your solar plexus. So let us bring some healing energy into this sponge, clearing your "gut level," which will aid digestion, and emotionally center you.

This method advances a sensation of being freed up. You will notice fullness of breath and a gut-level chaaa. The abdominal area tends to be very constricted and therefore experiences sensations ranging from tenderness to pain. Remember that whenever you find sensitive spots, your body is asking that you pay special attention to them. It is well worth the time to press into these points. As an added bonus, this exercise also enhances your breathing by releasing tension in your diaphragm, which is located directly above your solar plexus.

First, gently lay your hands over your solar plexus area for a minute or so. Feel into the area, press, and really tune into the underlying feelings. Often there is tension, a blockage, or outright pain here. In a clockwise direction, gradually allow your hands to descend from your solar plexus, increasing the pressure on your exhales. If you feel discomfort, breathe into it from within, and press into it. Direct the pressure downward to just below your belly button, then press back up to the base of your chest bone. Press, breathe, and feel.

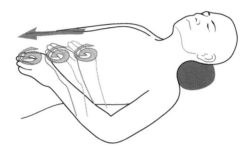

*Press clockwise from the sternum down just below the belly button*

Move the pressure clockwise, and as you do so, move your fingers in the same direction. Then apply pressure counterclockwise. Continue to press clockwise and counterclockwise until you feel an underlying sense of release.

Continue to do this until you simply do not want to press anymore—your body will tell you when it has had enough, and whether it needs a gentle or deeper touch. It is perfectly OK to press deeply, and it's OK to ease up.

This method facilitates letting go of the physical and emotional blockages you have in this area. Not only does it clear the gut, but it tends to clear the mind. After this practice, gently lay your hands over your solar plexus—breathe and feel it. Notice the sense of openness in the underlying area reflecting the vital circulation moving through you.

**EXERCISE:** *Moving Blocked Emotional Energy in the Gut*
This practice is a way to move blocked energy in your gut. It facilitates
your digestion and your overall emotional well-being.

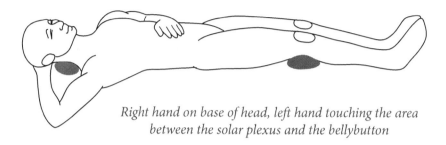

*Right hand on base of head, left hand touching the area
between the solar plexus and the bellybutton*

You will benefit most from this exercise when you are lying down.
Lay your right hand behind your head at the base of your skull. This
area when pressed relieves gastric and nervous tension. Place your left
hand over your solar plexus. Press into your solar plexus and breathe.
Enjoy the full-body soothing effect that pressing into these pressure
points along the back of the head and the solar plexus provide. Chaaa.

## Water
In Chinese medicine, the lower torso corresponds to the water
element. Your center of physical power is also located in this region—
your core. It is here that our strongest muscles connect from the thighs
into the lower torso. When this area stores tension, it gives us a sense
of being disjointed, or disconnected from our base. And when the
center is unstable, both the upper and lower body feel out of balance,
and our entire sense of well-being is off.

**EXERCISE:** *The Energetic Base*

The lower torso area of the body, your base, is also an energetic center. When you lay your hands on it and gently feel what is there, you connect to your energy base. This, in turn, balances you from the base up.

This is one of my favorite exercises. Start by lying down. Rest your right hand along the base of your skull. Gently press your left hand about two inches down from your belly button. Spread your fingers out along your pubic bone. Just gently feel if there is any tenderness, or simply enjoy how good this often feels.

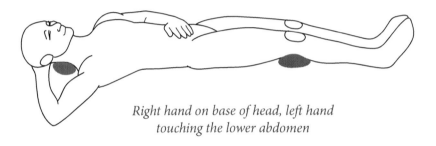

*Right hand on base of head, left hand
touching the lower abdomen*

Take a breath and breathe out into both hands, feeling your healing breath going into the back of your head and lower torso. Now take a full breath and send it down along the inside of your spine, into your pelvis, and then forward into your abdomen and chest. Do this three or four times, and then breathe normally. Be attentive to that tactile touch along the back of your head and down into the base of your torso. Stay with this feeling. This is a polarity practice in which you are simultaneously treating both areas of your body. Because there is polarized energy at both ends, the energy in your entire torso, head, and neck releases, bringing an overall sense of balance and wholeness. The secret is to feel it, and be it, because it really is you. Enjoy it.

## Dan Tien: A Secret to a Long Life

The dan tien point that we talked about earlier is located about two inches below the belly button. It is recognized in martial arts as the pivotal place of power and exertion. To be sure, it is worth it to acquaint yourself with your physical power center. A traditional Chinese medical longevity technique is to heat this point using a burning herb called moxa. This procedure often leaves a burn on the skin. Personally, I do not recommend this technique—it's a bit too radical for my tastes. I find that the combination of breathing, pressing, and keeping an open mind will produce similar results. When the energy in this region is moving, we stay strong. If it is blocked, our energetic center is off. Spending time in this lower abdominal region promotes a strong, physical sense of chaaa.

### EXERCISE: *Unlocking the Dan Tien*

This is one of my favorite ways to center myself. Do this when you have time to really let go, and do it as often as possible. Give yourself a comfortable space using pillows, towels, or whatever is necessary to chaaa and enjoy connecting with your life force.

Lying comfortably on your back, place your hands over your dan tien. Breathe in and out, focusing your exhales into this area. Now use both hands to slowly apply very soft pressure. Begin to lightly and lovingly press into any tender zones. Use the pressure of your hands to gently "ooze" energy into the tissues. Make sure you don't press or move around too much—stay gentle as you breathe into your hands.

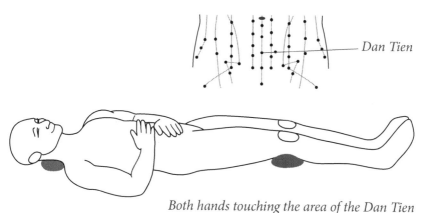

*Both hands touching the area of the Dan Tien*

The combination of breathing and pressing your dan tien creates movement in this part of your body. If there is no tension here, do this exercise for greater base energy awareness. This extremely satisfying exercise is a great way to chaaa, and it allows you to be in touch with your dan tien during the course of your day.

## Intrinsic Touch

We've already discussed the instinctive way many of us touch the pressure points in our foreheads when we feel anxiety or depression, but have you ever seen a person in shock press on the area just below the nose? I am always amazed at how we seem to intrinsically know to press on areas that correspond to our physical, emotional, and mental needs. The point just below the nose is an acupuncture point for resuscitation. It is used when people faint, or when they are in a sudden state of shock, or even when they are having a panic attack. This point will calm a person, and facilitate them from a physical, mental, or emotional crisis. Try pressing this area the next time you need some calming relief—if, that is, you don't do it instinctively! You can also begin any of the exercises in this book by pressing one or both of these pressure points to set a calm inner environment for the exercise.

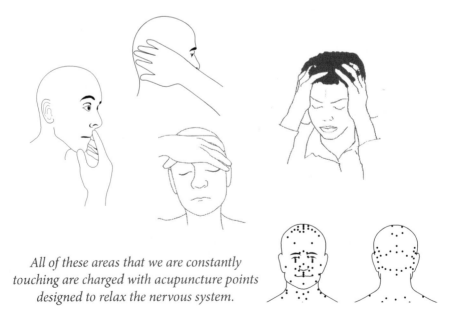

*All of these areas that we are constantly touching are charged with acupuncture points designed to relax the nervous system.*

Another area we instinctively touch when we are stressed is the temporal region. The temples and forehead are enriched with nerve endings and acupressure points. When they are pressed or touched, this stimulates the receptors on the skin, feeding nerve and energy stimulation to the brain, which results in an overall calming effect.

**EXERCISE:** *Full Body Earlobe Massage*

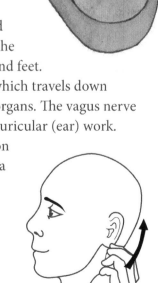

We fiddle with our ears. We are constantly pressing, rubbing, or touching them. This is certainly no random touch. The ears have connections. The World Health Organization currently recognizes 104 conditions that can be treated by stimulating pressure points in the ear, each of which corresponds to a body region. You can also access these pressure points for deep relaxation. From the perspective of Chinese medicine, the ear is a map of the entire body. The shape of the ear corresponds to a fetus in utero. The head represents the earlobe, and the ridge of the ear represents the back, buttocks, legs, and feet. Just under your ear is the vagus nerve, which travels down into the body and connects to the vital organs. The vagus nerve is the principal recipient of pressure in auricular (ear) work. This connection explains why pressing on ear points can be tantamount to getting a full body massage!

Starting at the earlobe, apply firm pressure moving up the outside of the ear, all the way to the apex, and then down onto the inner ridge. From there, follow the inner ridge of the ear all the way around to the hole of the ear itself.

If you find tender points, your ear is asking you to spend additional time there. Move slowly, and breathe as you massage along this path. Experiment with working one ear at a time, then both ears at the same time. For a minimal amount of energy, this daily massage pays huge, healthy dividends.

Once you've finished massaging your ears, try this add-on to your massage. Use your thumbs to press into your temples, and use your fingers to press into the pressure points along your forehead. To make this practice even more potent, project your exhalations slowly, into your hands and out into your temples and forehead.

## EXERCISE: *Shower Power*

The shower is a great place to randomly touch, explore, and make contact with yourself. The warm, moving water relaxes the muscles, creates a moist environment, and cleanses the body of old or stagnant energy. It also helps facilitate circulation and expands the muscles. The release of pressure you can feel by simply rubbing shampoo into your scalp is amazing. Water combined with pressure is a godsend!

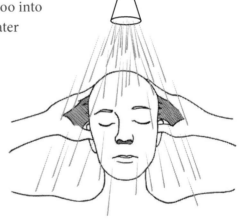

For this exercise, get into a warm shower. Once your body is warm and relaxed, spend a few minutes gently pressing or tapping around your body. Don't worry about doing this the wrong way or the right way—instead, just let your hands do their thing. Reach around to your upper back and lower neck regions, using your fingers to press into sensitive areas. Most people have some tenderness in these regions, so use your hands wisely and gently as you press and breathe into the muscles.

You can also do a variety of stretches as the warm water courses over your body. You can move congested or stagnant energy by beating on your chest, slapping your abdomen, and continuing down into your hips, groin, and legs. Even singing in the shower is a powerful tool for release—in fact, any kind of vocalization is great. Yodeling, singing, shouting, moaning, and humming are all wonderful ways to release your emotions, energy, and tension. Experiment with these and devise your own daily shower program. Go wild!

After showering, rub a towel briskly across your shoulders, upper back, and neck. The heat and friction stimulates circulation, particularly that of the lymphatic system.

## EXERCISE: *Bath Recharge*

As this book's main emphasis is on the yin approach, taking baths is obviously a "green light" activity. The warm water surrounding your body can send you into a deep, blissful chaaa state. So run a warm bath, and open your mind and body to this exercise.

As you sit in your bath, gently allow your hands to explore any tenderness or injury on your body. When you find a tender area, allow your fingers to rotate clockwise, then counter-clockwise, into that spot. Inhale quickly through the nose and exhale slowly out through the mouth. In your mind and body, project your exhalation out through your rotating fingers into the area of treatment. Once your body tells you you've spent enough time in one area, move on and explore further, stopping to breathe into any tender area you find. When you are finished, but still lying in the water, gently shake from within, feeling the internal waves of blissful energy as your body deeply breathes. Let go and chaaa!

## EXERCISE: *Yawning*

A yawn is quite different from a sigh. Yawning engages different muscles and nerve pathways, and it is also a great mouth and face stretch.

Most animals yawn. It's what we humans do first thing in the morning, and it helps wake us up, and get us ready for the day ahead. Many people think that yawning shows that a person is bored or disinterested. Research suggests the contrary. When you or someone else yawns, the body is saying, "I am relaxed and stimulated, at the same time."

A few good yawns change the way the brain functions, increasing its awareness, and relaxing the nervous system.

Try yawning three or four times when you feel nervous, anxious, or even tired. Students, you may want to try three or four yawns before exams to chaaa and help you turn on your brain juices.

## EXERCISE: *Vibrational Release*

Inhale through your nose. With your lips gently closed, blow through them so they vibrate like a running motor. It's the same thing we do to babies' cheeks when we want to have fun with them. This rumbling of the lips loosens the mouth and cheek muscles, and can produce a pleasant tingling sensation. It is also good for relaxing the face and even the voice.

Kissing is also a fun way to stimulate the sensory system of the entire body. A myriad of sensations can erupt from a great kiss. As a father of four children, I know that a kiss from daddy can somehow make a lot of minor injuries feel better. And, on the romantic side, we all know how much better it is when we kiss and make up. So, pucker up for longevity.

## Some Final Words on Alignment, Touch, and Breath

As we consciously breathe, touch, and move through our lives, with us comes the willful act of self-observation from a bird's-eye perspective. It is in loving the hungry, painful moments, observing and embracing the struggle, receiving strength through acceptance, and relishing in the beauty of it all that we arrive. And now that we are here, it is our duty to care for ourselves, and to enrich our lives with loving, healing practices. As you encounter life's joys and troubles, remember to align your body properly by holding yourself up toward the sky, use your healing touch and breath to resolve the conflicts within your body and mind, and most of all—chaaa.

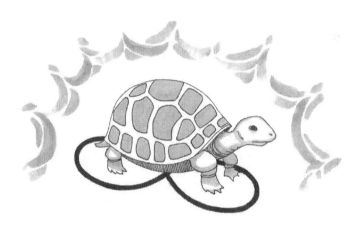

*Slow power wins the race in the truest sense!*

## Acknowledgments

I would like to wholeheartedly thank all of the people who helped in the process of creating this book. Steven Bendicson, Svetlana Petrowizky, Kristin and Edward, Sarah Irina Kovach, Donna and Sam Nevills, Marjorie Brownell and family, Gemini Ferrie, Kellee McQuinn, Barbara Dugan, Susie Anett, my niece Sarah, Artist Briget O. Rual, Matt Prine, Aalia Kazan Golden, and my beloved brother, Larry.

Thank you to my niece Ruby and her boyfriend Jimy. Special thanks to Jerome Dunn and Mara Corti. Thank you to Nurse Jane in the intensive care unit at UCLA, and to the rest of the medical team who helped my son.

Thanks to all of my teachers, students, and patients; to all my friends for showing up in the happy times and the sad times; and to the soccer players and dancers in my life. Thanks to my friends Ringo Starr, and his wife Barbara; to Jeff Lynne for being a friend, and fellow soccer fanatic; to Bob Dylan, and his family; and to George, Olivia, and Dahni Harrison.

Very special thanks to my children Vasant, Laila, Jahcai, Hyacinth, and my stepson Kjel, who in their process of growth, have shown me great purpose and joy, and who have always reminded me to have fun!

And very special thanks to Katherine Mestalos Kearney, for being a powerful inspiration with her display of great healing after a serious spinal cord injury, and for being the mother of my two oldest children.

I give my thanks to Heidi Crum for giving birth to my two youngest children; to my siblings, Larry, Paul, Raymond, Brian, Noel, Philomena, and Elizabeth; and to all my nephews and nieces. Thank you for being my family and friends.

## About the Author

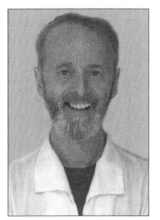

A native of Ireland, Dr. Kearney immigrated to Australia when he was 13 years old. In 1975, after receiving a diploma from the Acupuncture College of Australia, Dr. Kearney joined the faculty there and began lecturing in Sydney, Melbourne, Adelaide, and Brisbane. During this time, he also attended the New South Wales College of Naturopathy and Osteopathy in Sydney.

As one of the few qualified teachers of Chinese medicine in the late 1970s, Dr. Kearney was invited by the California Acupuncture College to become head of their acupuncture department (the second institution of its kind accredited in California).

At this time he was instrumental in the implementation of Chinese medicine on the West Coast. During the course of his studies at the International College of Chinese Medicine and at the Acupuncture College of Australia, he studied under the tutelage of Dr. Van Buren, master acupuncturist and osteopath, and Dr. Russell Jewell. Both taught him the integration of energetic and physical medicine. In 1986, Dr. Kearney received a doctorate of Chinese medicine from the California Acupuncture College.

His search for alternative healing reached a spiritual level when he became a monk, and practiced meditation and celibacy for five years. This pursuit brought him to the U.S. Through his practice as a monk, and as a doctor of energetic medicine, he developed his own unique style of breathing and meditation, which is the basis for the breathing practices he teaches.

Over a period of 15 years, Dr. Kearney traveled nationally and internationally, with various musical acts. He is recognized with special acknowledgments on Bob Dylan's album, *Knocked Out and Loaded*, as well as George Harrison's album, *Cloud Nine*.

His transformative self-healing workshop, "Chaaa Healing," has been a popular healing tool for decades. The course has been taught extensively, and has helped thousands of people gain the practical knowledge presented more extensively in this book. The video, *Power Healing*, that paired with his workshop features an opening interview with Ringo Starr, who attests to the value of Dr. Kearney's breath work.

For the last 36 years, he has maintained a private practice in West Los Angeles, and has experienced success with a wide variety of patient cases, including rehabilitating patients after severe spinal cord trauma.

When he is not practicing meditation or medicine, Dr. Kearney is most likely to be found on the soccer field, working in his garden, jumping on a trampoline, or dancing on the dance floor.

## Bibliography

Edlund, Matthew, MD. *The Power of Rest: Why Sleep Alone Is Not Enough*. New York: Harper One, 2010.

Farhi Donna. *The Breathing Book: Good Health and Vitality*. New York: Henry Holt, 1996.

Fried, Robert, PhD. *The Breath Connection: How to Reduce Psychosomatic and Stress Related Disorders With Easy-To-Do Breathing Exercises*. Insight Books, 1990.

Kearney, David, OMD. *Power Healing*, DVD. Produced by David Kearney, directed by Charles Lange. Los Angeles, 1998.

Lipton, Bruce H., PhD. *The Biology of Belief: Unleashing the Power of Consciousness, Matter and Miracles*. Hay House, 2005.

Sue, Steven K. DDS, Designer of the Nose Breathe mouthpiece. Honolulu, HI.

Missri, Jose C., MD and Alexander, Sydney, MD. Hyperventilation Syndrome, A Brief Review. *Journal of the American Medical Association*, Nov 3, 1978, Vol. 240, No. 19.

## Chaaa Endorsement

The flight-fight stress response enabled our ancestors to escape danger for tens of thousands of years, but in modern times this same survival system is killing us through stress-related diseases. The danger has moved inside our minds and appears as fear, worry, anger, depression, and anxiety. David Kearney's powerful chaaa practice brings harmony back to mind and body, thereby making stress once again our friend.

Ronald L. Peters, MD, MPH
MindBody Medicine Center
Scottsdale, Arizona

Made in the USA
Middletown, DE
07 October 2018